Clinical Gynaecology:
A Quick-Reference Guide

Fourth edition

Editors
T F Kruger
M H Botha

Clinical Gynaecology: A Quick-Reference Guide

First edition 1993
Second edition 2001
Third edition 2007
Fourth edition 2011

ISBN 978 07021 86684

© Juta and Company Ltd, 2011
1st floor, Sunclare Building
21 Dreyer Street
Claremont
7708

Project management: Johanna Breakey
Editor: Annette de Villiers
Proofreader: Pat Hanekom
Illustrator: Carol Lochner
Cover design: Pumphaus Design Studio
Typesetting by Mckore Graphics

CONTENTS

SECTION 4

UROGYNAECOLOGY

SECTION 1 | Oncology (Benign and malignant diseases)

1 | Diseases of the vagina

B G Lindeque

(See Chapter 7 of *Clinical Gynaecology*, 4th edition for more detailed information.)

CLASSIFICATION

There are several diseases which can occur in the vagina, either as *de novo* conditions or as part of disorders affecting other parts of the genital tract.

Table 1.1 Diseases of the vagina

Vaginitis	Postmenopausal atrophic vaginitis Emphysematous vaginitis Toxic shock syndrome
Cystic lesions	Epidermal cysts Congenital cysts Endometriosis
Solid tumours	Condylomata acuminata Polyps Leiomyomata
Vaginal adenosis	
Premalignant lesions	VAIN I, II and III
Malignant lesions	Invasive squamous carcinoma Adenocarcinoma Melanoma Sarcoma DES-related malignancies Secondary malignancies

MALIGNANT LESIONS

Primary vaginal malignancies are rare and constitute 1 percent of gynaecological cancers. As a general rule, a vaginal malignancy should be regarded as a metastasis until proven otherwise.

Table 1.2 FIGO staging of vaginal carcinoma

Stage I	Carcinoma limited to the vaginal wall.
Stage II	Involvement of subvaginal tissues, not reaching the pelvic wall.
Stage III	Extension to the pelvic wall.
Stage IV	Extension beyond the true pelvis; involvement of the mucosa of the bladder or rectum.

NOTES:

2 | Diseases of the vulva

T Smith

(See Chapter 8 of *Clinical Gynaecology*, 4th edition for more detailed information.)

DERMATOLOGICAL CONDITIONS

- **Dermatitis** may be caused by contact with an irritant, such as laundry detergents, toilet paper, deodorants, dusting powders, lubricants and spermicides
- **Lichen planus** may cause redness, soreness and burning associated with raw areas of skin
- **Psoriasis** can affect the vulva alone.

INFECTIONS

- **Candidiasis** is caused by an overgrowth of yeast-like fungi called *Candida albicans* and may be treated with local or systemic imidazole derivatives
- **Herpes simplex** causes painful shallow vesicles that may become secondarily infected and antiviral medications can help reduce the duration and severity of an outbreak
- **Condylomata acuminata** (genital warts) are commonly associated with human papillomavirus types 6 and 11. A vaccine may be important in decreasing the incidence of warts in the female population
- **Syphilis** is caused by the spirochaete *Treponema pallidum*. Recommended treatment is with benzathine penicillin G, 2.4 million units intramuscularly, or erythromycin 500 mg, qid for three weeks if the patient is allergic
- **Lymphogranuloma venereum** is caused by *Chlamydia trachomatis*. Doxycycline or erythromycin should be given orally for at least three weeks
- **Molluscum contagiosum** appear as dome-shaped lumps, 1–2 mm in diameter with tiny dimples in their centre, and contain a cheese-like substance.

BENIGN LESIONS

Bartholin's cysts occur when ducts of the Bartholin's glands are obstructed at their vestibular orifice and the obstruction results in subsequent cystic dilatation of the duct. A Bartholin's abscess is an acute process often associated with *Neisseria gonorrhoeae* infection, although it may be related to staphylococci or anaerobic organisms. The affected Bartholin's gland should be marsupialised.

PIGMENTATION DISORDERS OF THE VULVA

Hypopigmented conditions
- Vitiligo
- Albinism
- Leukoderma.

Hyperpigmented lesions
- Freckles (ephelides)
- Lentigo simplex
- Naevomelanocytic naevi
- Pre-malignant and malignant growths.

NON-NEOPLASTIC EPITHELIAL DISORDERS

- Lichen sclerosus
- Squamous cell hyperplasia
- Other dermatoses.

MALIGNANCIES OF THE VULVA

Malignant tumours of the vulva constitute 3–5 percent of all gynaecological malignancies, and invasive squamous cell carcinoma constitutes approximately 80 percent of all primary vulvar malignant tumours. The remaining 20 percent are basal cell carcinomas, malignant melanomas, sarcomas and carcinomas of Bartholin's gland or sweat glands.

3 | Vulvodynia

J Tankel, P F Kruger

(See Chapter 9 of *Clinical Gynaecology*, 4th edition for more detailed information.)

TERMINOLOGY AND CLASSIFICATION

"Vulvar discomfort, most often described as burning pain, occurring in the absence of relevant visible findings or a specific, clinically identifiable, neurological disorder." (As classified by the ISSVD.)

The International Society for the Study of Vulvovaginal Disease (ISSVD) further classifies vulvodynia as follows:

- Generalised vulvodynia
  - Provoked (sexual, nonsexual or both)
  - Unprovoked
  - Mixed.
- Localised vulvodynia
  - Provoked (sexual, nonsexual or both) also known as provoked vestibulodynia/Vulvar Vestibulitis Syndrome
  - Unprovoked
  - Mixed.

AETIOLOGY AND PATHOGENESIS

The pathogenesis of vulvodynia is unknown.

DIAGNOSTIC EVALUATION

- The diagnosis of vulvodynia is one of exclusion. A thorough history should characterise the patient's pain, identifying the onset, duration, location associated symptoms, alleviating and aggravating factors.
- Cotton swab testing (Fig 3.1) is used to identify areas of localised pain and to classify the areas where there is mild, moderate, or severe pain.

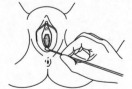

Figure 3.1 Cotton swab testing.

TREATMENT

Treatment of generalised vulvodynia

A multi-disciplinary treatment approach includes:
- Topical preparations
- Oral "pain-blocking" medications
- Nerve blocks
- Physiotherapy (pelvic floor therapy)
- Psychotherapy.

Treatment of provoked vestibulodynia

Again, initial treatment includes
- Education, counselling as well as vulvar self-care
- A multi-disciplinary and stepwise approach
- Medical treatment
- Physical therapy
- Psychotherapy
- Surgery is an option in this group.

4 | Carcinoma of the cervix

B G Lindeque

(See Chapter 41 in *Clinical Gynaecology*, 4th edition for more detailed information.)

INTRODUCTION

- Cervical carcinoma remains the most common gynaecological malignancy in SA
- Cervical cancers pass through a premalignant precursor phase which can be detected and treated.

EPIDEMIOLOGY AND AETIOLOGY

- HPV infection
- HPV types may best be divided into low-risk and high-risk groups
- HPV is predominantly, but not exclusively, a sexually transmitted virus
- When host factors are favourable, integration of viral DNA into host DNA occurs, leading to the formation of dysplastic cells. This process is termed "cervical carcinogenesis"
- Genetic: The cellular "mopup protein" p53 has been demonstrated to be deficient in patients with cervical cancer
- Infectious: HIV
- Coital:
  - Age at first coitus is the next important risk factor
  - Coitus with multiple sexual partners
- Cigarette smoking: This is associated with a twofold increase in the risk.

PREMALIGNANT LESIONS OF THE CERVIX

- Histologically the premalignant lesion is termed "cervical intraepithelial neoplasia"
- Subclassified into the three grades of CIN 1, CIN 2 and CIN 3:
  - CIN 1, dysplastic cells in the lower third of the cervical epithelium
  - CIN 2, dysplastic cells are present in the lower two-thirds
  - CIN 3, in the full thickness of the epithelium.

PRIMARY PREVENTION OF CERVICAL CANCER

- HPV vaccines against high-risk HPV 16/18
- Anti-smoking campaigns
- Campaigns to promote good sexual health.

SECONDARY PREVENTION OF CERVICAL CANCER

- Screening for premalignant lesions
- Screening for HPV is an option
  - It is available but is expensive
  - Cannot be used as primary screening in patients younger than 30
- Conventional cytology to screen for cytological abnormality:
  - Squamous intraepithelial lesion low-grade (LSIL) (equivalent to the histological diagnosis of CIN 1 and/or HPV)
  - Squamous intraepithelial lesion high-grade (HSIL) (equivalent to the histological diagnosis of CIN 2 and 3)
  - ASC (atypical squamous cells) that may have undetermined significance or may possibly favour premalignancy.

MANAGEMENT OF PREMALIGNANT LESIONS

- LSIL on cytology followed six to twelve months with repeat smears
- Persistent LSIL present for more than a year is an indication for referral
- HSIL smears should be referred
- LSIL lesions may be treated with cryotherapy
- LLETZ may offer a "one-stop" diagnosis and treatment visit for HSIL on cytology
- Vaginal hysterectomy may sometimes be offered as definitive therapy for CIN 2 and CIN 3.

INVASIVE SQUAMOUS CARCINOMA OF THE CERVIX

Clinical presentation
- Asymptomatic in the early stages
- Abnormal vaginal bleeding
- Offensive vaginal discharge
- Pain
- Weight loss
- Vesicovaginal or rectovaginal fistulae.

Diagnosis and staging
- Histological diagnosis is mandatory
- Cervical carcinoma is staged clinically according FIGO.

Management
- Surgery is applicable to Stages I and IIa
- Radiotherapy/chemotherapy can be utilised in all stages.

5 | Malignancies of the uterine corpus

G C du Toit

(See Chapter 43 in *Clinical Gynaecology*, 4th edition for more detailed information.)

Primary malignancies of the uterine body (corpus) are:
- Endometrial carcinoma
- Sarcomas
- Carcinosarcomas.

ENDOMETRIAL CARCINOMA

Aetiology
- An oestrogen-dependant tumour in the majority of cases
- Unopposed, prolonged oestrogen stimulation of the endometrium
- A small group (15 percent) of the endometrial carcinomas develops in the absence of oestrogen stimulation.

Epidemiology
- Obesity
- Nulliparous patients
- Family history of endometrial carcinoma
- Delayed menopause
- Exogenous unopposed oestrogen, endogenous unopposed oestrogen (anovulation)
- Medical disorders such as hypertension and diabetes.

Pathology
- Adenocarcinoma
- Adenocarcinoma with squamous metaplasia
- Adenosquamous carcinoma
- Other (clear cell carcinoma, papillary serous adenocarcinoma).

Patterns of spread
- Directly into the myometrium
- Lymphatic spread to the pelvic lymph nodes as well as the para-aortic lymph nodes
- Haematogenous spread occurs late to the lungs, liver, skeletal bones and, rarely, the brain.

Clinical presentation
- Postmenopausal bleeding
- Vaginal discharge
- Pain is a late symptom.

Diagnosis and special investigations
- Clinical assessment
- Transvaginal ultrasound (for endometrial lining)
- Histological diagnosis obtained by hysteroscopy or dilatation and curettage or endometrial sampling.

Treatment
Surgery
- Total abdominal hysterectomy, bilateral salpingo-oopherectomy and peritoneal lavage
- In certain selected cases, pelvic lymph node dissection may be indicated
- Radical hysterectomy if cervix is involved.

Radiation therapy
- Depending on risk factors identified by surgical resected specimen, radiotherapy may be indicated
- Whole pelvic radiotherapy and/or radiotherapy to the vaginal vault may be indicated.

Chemotherapy
- Hormonal and chemotherapy may be indicated in cases with metastatic disease.

Follow-up
- After completion of the therapy (surgery and/or radiotherapy), patients should be meticulously followed up for recurrence of disease or complications of radiotherapy.

Survival
- In most cases with endometrial carcinoma present in stage I and depending on the stage of disease the survival is excellent.

UTERINE SARCOMAS
Aetiology
- Previous pelvic radiotherapy is associated with an increased risk for the development of uterine sarcomas.

Classification
- Uterine sarcomas are classified according to histopathological cell type
- Carcinosarcomas refers to mixed Müllerian tumours and these tumours consist of a malignant soft tissue (stromal) component as well as a malignant epithelial carcinoma component
- The most common sarcomas are leiomyosarcomas, carcinosarcomas and endometrial stromal sarcomas (ESS).

Clinical features
- Lower abdominal mass
- Postmenopausal bleeding
- Peak incidence varies between 45 and 55 years.

Treatment
- Primary surgical with tailored postoperative adjuvant therapy.

6 | Postmenopausal bleeding (PMB)

F H van der Merwe

(See Chapter 42 in *Clinical Gynaecology*, 4th edition for more detailed information.)

Postmenopausal bleeding is defined as any bleeding from the female genital tract in the appropriate aged woman (refer to Chapters 29 and 42) not using hormonal therapy at least six months after the cessation of menstruation **or** acyclical vaginal bleeding in a postmenopausal woman on hormonal therapy. Principle: although there are many causes for postmenopausal bleeding, malignancy must always be ruled out, especially endometrial carcinoma.

AETIOLOGY

Systemic
- Bleeding disorders
  - Thrombocytopenia, Von Willebrand's
  - Anticoagulants
- Exogenous oestrogens
  - Hormone therapy
  - Natural products, for example soy
- Endogenous oestrogens
  - Peripheral conversion of androgens
  - Oestrogen-producing tumours.

Local
- Benign
  - Vulval dystrophies
  - Vulval dermatitis
  - Vulval trauma
  - Atrophic vaginitis
  - Vaginal trauma
  - Vaginal inflammation
  - Vaginal polyps
  - Cervical polyps
  - Cervicitis
  - Cervical trauma
  - Endometrial polyps
  - Endometritis
  - Endometrial atrophy
  - Uterine fibroids.

- Malignant
    - Premalignant
    - Vulval carcinoma
    - Vaginal carcinoma
    - Cervical carcinoma
    - Endometrial hyperplasia
    - Endometrial carcinoma
    - Uterine sarcomas
    - Fallopian tube carcinoma
    - Secondary tumours.

HISTORY AND CLINICAL EXAMINATION

History
- Elicit the exact nature of the bleeding
- Possible systemic causes can be excluded
- Medication
- Associated symptoms
- Factors associated with an increased risk of endometrial carcinoma and hyperplasia should be considered.

Examination
- General examination
- Abdominal examination
- Vulva and vagina
- Cervix
- Uterus and adnexae
- Rectum.

FURTHER INVESTIGATIONS

- Side-room investigations: Urinalysis, faecal occult blood, haemoglobin, cervical cytology
- Pipelle endometrial sampling
- Ultrasound (transvaginal)
- Saline infusion sonohysterography (SIS)
- Hysteroscopy and biopsy.

7 | Ovarian tumours

B G Lindeque

(See Chapter 44 in *Clinical Gynaecology*, 4th edition for more detailed information.)

INTRODUCTION

- Approximately 75 percent of all ovarian tumours are benign and 25 percent are malignant
- The peak incidence of benign ovarian tumours is between 20 and 45 years
- Malignant ovarian tumours occur mostly between 45 and 65 years
- 80 percent of malignant epithelial tumours are found in postmenopausal women.

FUNCTIONAL BENIGN CYSTS OF THE OVARY

- **Follicle cysts** are usually solitary with a smooth surface and a clear liquid content
- **Theca lutein cysts** are multicystic and may be associated with a hydatidiform mole, or may follow induction of ovulation
- **Corpus luteum cysts** must be at least 2 cm in diameter and usually measure 7–8 cm.

Ultrasound criteria usually associated with a benign cyst are:
- Unilocularity (only one cyst)
- Clear contents (echo-free contents)
- Thin cyst walls
- Smooth cyst walls (no papillary growths on the cyst walls)
- Size less than 8 cm in diameter
- Unilaterality
- No ascitic fluid present.

Complications of cysts
- Persisting cysts
- Rupture and bleeding
- Torsion.

NONFUNCTIONAL BENIGN CYSTS OF THE OVARY

- **Polycystic ovaries and hyperthecosis**: the ovaries may markedly enlarge and appear tumour-like

- **Endometriomata**: ovarian involvement by endometriosis may cause surface lesions and also ovarian cystic endometriosis, called endometriomata
- **Para-ovarian cysts** arise from embryological remnants of the Wolffian duct within the two layers of the broad ligament
- **Residual ovary syndrome**: functioning ovary may be stuck to the vaginal vault or peritoneal surfaces after hysterectomy, be partly enclosed by adhesions, and cysts and pseudocysts may form with ovulation
- **Ovarian remnant syndrome**: presence of ovarian tissue after a presumed bilateral oophorectomy.

TUMOUR-LIKE CONDITIONS OF THE OVARY

- **Pregnancy luteoma** is composed of solid nodules of luteinised cells
- **Massive oedema** of the ovary is usually unilateral, and may be as much as 30 cm.

OVARIAN NEOPLASMS

Classification of ovarian neoplasms is according to the tissue of origin:
- Epithelial tumours
- Stromal tumours
- Germ cell tumours
- Metastatic tumours.

Features suggestive of malignancy on pelvic ultrasound include:
- Solid or cystic and solid mass
- Multilocular cysts
- Thick cyst walls
- Papillary growths on inner or outer surfaces
- Bilaterality
- Ascitic fluid present.

MANAGEMENT OF EPITHELIAL OVARIAN CARCINOMA

All stages require initial surgical staging and debulking:
- Stages Ia and Ib: surgical resection is adequate, especially in cases with well-differentiated tumours
- Patients in Stages Ia and Ib with poorly differentiated tumours, and those in Stage Ic, will require chemotherapy. Such treatment is given for a limited number of cycles and frequently with a single agent, and the outlook is favourable
- Stages II, III and IV require tumour reduction followed by chemotherapy for six to eight cycles over a period of six to eight months. Cisplatin-based combination chemotherapy is most widely used.

Table 7.1 Surgical staging classification for ovarian carcinomas (FIGO 1988)

Stage I:
Growth limited to the ovaries.

Stage II:
Growth involving one or both ovaries with pelvic extension.

Stage III:
Tumour involving one or both ovaries with peritoneal implants outside the pelvis and/or positive retroperitoneal or inguinal nodes; superficial liver metastases equals Stage III; tumour is limited to the true pelvis but with histologically proven malignant extension to small bowel or omentum.

Stage IV:
Extension to other pelvic tissues. Growth involving one or both ovaries with distant metastases. If pleural effusion is present, there must be positive cytology to allot a case to Stage IV; parenchymal liver metastases equal Stage IV.

NOTES:

8 | Gestational trophoblastic disease (GTD)

M Moodley

(See Chapter 46 in *Clinical Gynaecology*, 4th edition for more detailed information.)

INTRODUCTION

Gestational Trophoblastic Disease (GTD) comprises a spectrum of abnormal proliferation of the trophoblast. The term Gestational Trophoblastic Neoplasia (GTN) can be used for all persistent GTDs. These conditions produce human chorionic gonadotropin (hCG) and are managed medically with chemotherapy. Surgery has a limited but important secondary role.

CLASSIFICATION

World Health Organisation (WHO) classification of GTD includes:
- Hydatidiform mole (HM):
  - Complete
  - Partial
- Invasive mole (IM)
- Choriocarcinoma (CC)
- Placental trophoblastic tumour (PSTT)
- Epitheloid trophoblastic tumour
- Miscellaneous trophoblastic lesions:
  - Exaggerated placental site
  - Placental site nodule or plaque
  - Unclassified trophoblastic lesions.

RISK FACTORS

- Age (higher at young and old spectrum of fertility)
- Race (Asian)
- Blood Group B
- Cigarette smoking
- Past molar pregnancy.

CLINICAL FEATURES

- Vaginal bleeding (grape-like vesicles)
- Hyperemesis gravidarum
- Early onset pre-eclampsia
- Hyperthyroidism

- Uterus larger than expected (50 percent cases)
- Vaginal metastases.

DIAGNOSIS

Combination of clinical, biochemical and radiological features.

WORK-UP

Investigations necessary for confirmation and work-up:
1. Blood tests:
   - Full blood count, coagulation profile (INR/PTT), renal function (U/E), TFT, Rhesus, hCG (quantative), crossmatch.

2. Radiological tests:
   - Chest X-ray
   - Ultrasound pelvis and abdomen
   - Doppler colour flow of the uterus to exclude invasive mole
   - CT/MRI of the brain only if the chest X-ray demonstrates lung metastases.

MANAGEMENT

Non-invasive molar pregnancy
- Resuscitation
- Suction curettage under ultrasound guidance
- Follow up: weekly hCG estimations
- Contraception 12 months.

Post hydatidiform GTN

GTN may be diagnosed when any of the following criteria are met:
1. When the plateau of hCG levels lasts for four measurements (days 1, 7, 14 and 21) over a period of three weeks or longer
2. When there is a rise in hCG level for three weekly consecutive measurements (days 1, 7 and 14) or longer, over a period of at least two weeks or more
3. When the hCG level remains elevated for six months or more
4. When there is histological diagnosis of choriocarcinoma.

Table 8.1 The FIGO anatomical staging

Stage	Criteria
I	Disease confined to the uterus
II	Disease outside the uterus, but limited to genital structures
III	Disease extending to the lungs with or without genital tract spread
IV	All other metastatic sites

Management of GTN

- Patients are scored according to the FIGO 2000 staging system
- Low-risk patients have a score of 6 or less. High-risk patients have a score of 7 or more. Low-risk patients are treated with single-agent methotrexate or Dactinomycin followed with folinic acid rescue
- Patients with a score of >7 are treated with combination chemotherapy
- Patients with histologically confirmed placental trophoblastic tumours (PSTT) are treated with hysterectomy and combination chemotherapy.

Surgery

The indications for surgery include:

- Suction curettage under ultrasound guidance for a non-invasive molar pregnancy
- Hysterectomy for disease confined to the uterus in women who have completed child-bearing
- Resection of isolated chemotherapy-resistant nodules, for example thoracotomy, craniotomy
- Laparotomy for bowel or urinary tract obstruction
- Oophorectomy for torsion of ovarian cysts
- Persistent PSTT.

Haemorrhage

Management of significant haemorrhage from vaginal metastases:

- Insertion of urinary catheter
- Vaginal packing with gauze
- Resuscitation
- Selective angiographic localisation and embolisation of pelvic vessels if vaginal packing is unsuccessful
- Ligation of the internal iliac artery if embolisation fails.

Management of uterine or intra-abdominal haemorrhage:

- Resuscitation and angiographic embolisation of the feeding vessels
- Ligation of the internal iliac artery is rarely indicated
- Hysterectomy is indicated if embolisation fails.

SECTION 2 | General gynaecology

9 | Pelvic inflammatory disease

K Coetsee, F Paruk

(See Chapter 13 in *Clinical Gynaecology*, 4th edition for more detailed information.)

DIAGNOSIS

Table 9.1 Clinical diagnosis of pelvic inflammatory disease

A triad of:
- Lower abdominal pain/tenderness (dull/aching)
- Cervical excitation tenderness
- Adnexal and uterine tenderness (unilateral/bilateral).

Plus one of the following should be present:
- Temperature >38.3 °C
- Abundant white blood cells (WBS) on saline microscopy of vaginal secretions
- Mucopurulent discharge from the cervix
- Erythrocyte sedimentation rate (ESR) >15 mm/hour
- Elevated C-Reactive Protein (CPR).

Table 9.2 Differential diagnosis

- Ectopic pregnancy
- Appendicitis
- Pyelonephritis
- Torsion of an ovarian cyst
- Rupture of an ovarian cyst
- Haemorrhage into an ovarian cyst
- Bleeding corpus luteum cyst
- Ruptured endometrioma
- Diverticulitis
- Amoebiasis
- Regional lymphadenitis
- Typhoid
- Gastroenteritis
- Mittelschmertz pain
- Renal colic.

CLASSIFICATION

In the context of the Gainesville Classification, the therapeutic goals are as follows:

Stage I   Eliminate symptoms and infectivity

Stage II   Preservation of Fallopian tube function

Stage III   Preservation of ovarian function

Stage IV   Preservation of the patient's life.

In the context of the Gainesville Classification, the treatments are as follows:

Stage I   Outpatient treatment with oral antibiotics

Stage II   Inpatient treatment with parenteral antibiotics

Stage III   Inpatient treatment with parenteral antibiotics (Tripple therapy) and surgery if no improvement after 48 hours

Stage IV   Laparotomy and triple antibiotics.

SEQUELAE OF PID

- **Recurrence of PID**: This occurs in 25 percent of patients
- **Infertility:** The occlusive tubal damage caused by PID is responsible for infertility
- **Ectopic pregnancy:** The incidence of ectopic pregnancy increases by a factor of seven following an episode of PID
- **Chronic pain:** This occurs in 20 percent of patients
- **Psychological sequelae**
- **Mortality:** This occurs occasionally in the situation of severe disease manifesting with septic shock and/or multiorgan dysfunction syndrome.

TREATMENT

Outpatient management

Outpatient treatment should be effective for mild to moderate disease. As the microbiological aetiology is usually unknown at the time of the initial assessment, it is important to treat for gonococcal and chlamydial infection.

Inpatient treatment for PID

General measures

- Hydration of patient with intravenous infusion and correct antibiotic regime
- Analgesia
- Regular monitoring of blood pressure, pulse rate, respiratory rate, temperature and urine output
- Serial assessment of systemic, abdominal and pelvic signs.

Medical therapy

At Tygerberg Hospital the following regime is used:

- Ampicillin (Penbrittin) 1 gram every 6 hours
- Gentamycin [Garamycin ±240 mg daily (5mg/kg daily IV)]
- Metronidazole (Flagyl) 500 mg every 8 hours.
- Surgical intervention
- Generalised peritonitis
- Pelvic absesses.

A laparotomy is indicated in the following situations:

- Generalised peritonitis
- Tubo-ovarian abscess which does not respond to appropriate antimicrobial therapy within 48 hours
- A pelvic abscess, which is pointing into the vagina, rectum or abdominal wall
- Uncertainty about the diagnosis.

10 | Ectopic pregnancy

T Matsaseng

(See Chapter 14 in *Clinical Gynaecology*, 4th edition for more detailed information.)

DEFINITION

An ectopic pregnancy occurs when the developing blastocyst implants anywhere other than in the endometrial lining of the uterine cavity. The incidence of ectopic pregnancy is approximately 2 percent in the general population.

RISK FACTORS

Knowledge of the risk factors for ectopic pregnancy assists in identifying patients at risk and in making an early diagnosis, hence an early treatment. This allows the clinician to consider a more conservative approach.

Extrauterine pregnancies contribute substantially to maternal mortality in all parts of the world.

Table 10.1 (14.1) Risk factors for ectopic pregnancy

1. Previous tubal surgery
2. Infertility and assisted reproduction
3. Confirmed previous genital infection
4. Previous miscarriage
5. Previous induced abortion
6. Past or current smoker
7. Age 40 years and older
8. Sterilisation
9. Previous ectopic pregnancy
10. Documented tubal pathology
11. Sexual promiscuity
12. Diethylstilboestrol exposure

PATHOLOGY

The natural progression of a tubal pregnancy is as follows:

- Tubal rupture with severe intra-abdominal haemorrhage
- Tubal abortion
- Spontaneous resolution
- Chronic ectopic pregnancy.

DIAGNOSIS

The classic triad of symptoms associated with ectopic pregnancy includes:

■ Amenorrhoea or a recent irregular menstrual period
■ Vaginal bleeding
■ Abdominal pain.

The clinical presentation can easily be confused with a miscarriage. When clinical features are equivocal, pelvic ultrasonography is most valuable in identifying an intrauterine pregnancy.

Human chorionic gonadotropin (hCG)

Urine pregnancy tests detect only higher levels of hCG. A negative test, therefore, does not exclude an early ectopic pregnancy. This must be followed by a highly sensitive blood hCG test.

The introduction of quantitative β-hCG and transvaginal ultrasound has improved diagnostic capabilities.

MANAGEMENT

In most cases, surgery remains the first choice in the management of an ectopic pregnancy. However, early diagnosis allows the options of medical management.

Unruptured ectopic pregnancy

■ Medical therapy with methotrexate is indicated in patients with no evidence of rupture, β-hCG levels $\leq 3\ 000$ IU/L and no fetal cardiac activity on ultrasound
■ Surgical management of an unruptured ectopic pregnancy is indicated where the likelihood of success of non-surgical, treatment is remote
■ Surgery is indicated if a β-hCG level of $>3\ 000$ IU/L and fetal cardiac activity on ultrasound.

Ruptured ectopic pregnancy

Massive haemorrhage is practically defined as symptomatic bleeding that requires an emergency intervention to save the patient's life. The aim should be quick resuscitation and transfer to the operating theatre for surgery to stop the bleeding.

Basic principles for the surgery of a ruptured – ectopic pregnancy

1. Obtain good exposure of the pelvis through an adequate abdominal access.
2. Do not waste valuable time in trying to clear blood from the peritoneal cavity.
3. Identify the site of active bleeding and stop the bleeding initially with an arterial clamp.

4. Once the bleeding has been stopped temporarily, the anaesthetic team should achieve haemodynamic stability while the surgeon performs a salpingectomy.

ADVANCED ABDOMINAL PREGNANCY

Advanced abdominal pregnancy is a rare condition, the frequency of which is difficult to establish accurately. Estimates of its incidence vary between (1 : 402 and 1 : 50 820) deliveries. It is associated with a high perinatal mortality (40–95 percent), a high rate of congenital malformations (30–90 percent), and a maternal mortality rate of 0.5–18 percent.

R C Pattinson, L C Snyman

(See Chapter 15 in *Clinical Gynaecology*, 4th edition for more detailed information.)

Miscarriage is one of the most common gynaecological problems a medical practitioner will encounter. It is still one of the major causes of maternal death in South Africa. Septic incomplete abortions remain a significant contributor to maternal morbidity and mortality, despite a liberal termination of pregnancy Act.

DEFINITION

- An abortion: the ending of a pregnancy before the fetus is viable
- According to South African law, viability is defined as 6 months (26 weeks) after conception – in other words, 28 weeks after the last menstrual period.

CLINICAL PRESENTATION AND MANAGEMENT

Threatened abortion

- Light vaginal bleeding with or without backache or abdominal pain
- Cervix is closed
- Fetus is alive.

Management: conservative

Inevitable abortion

- Increasing pain and vaginal bleeding
- Uterus may be tender
- Dilatation of the cervix.

Management

- If shocked, resuscitation.
- In the first trimester, a suction curettage/manual vacuum aspiration is performed
- In the second trimester, adequate pain relief and oxytocin should be administered during the abortion process and the patient should be allowed first to abort spontaneously. This is then followed by a vacuum aspiration of the retained products of conception
- If the placenta is aborted completely, which often occurs only after 16–18 weeks, an evacuation can be omitted.

Incomplete abortion

- Passing of products of conception, whether these are amniotic fluid, placental tissue or the fetus
- History that she has passed something and the cramps became less painful
- On examination, the uterus is smaller than expected for the gestational age
- The cervix is open and products of conception can often be felt through the cervical os.

Management

- Any retained products should be removed by an ovum forceps during the initial evaluation of the patient
- The evacuation can be performed by manual vacuum aspiration if the uterus is not bigger than 12 weeks' size, or surgical curettage can be done irrespective of the actual gestational age.

Complete abortion

The abortion is complete and the uterus empty. Vaginal or abdominal ultrasound is often helpful in the diagnosis.

If the pregnancy is beyond 16–18 weeks, the whole fetus and placenta can be expelled, which is referred to as a complete abortion. This can only be diagnosed if the clinician has seen the products of conception him- or herself and confirmed that they are complete.

Management

- In 90 percent of cases of an early abortion (less than six weeks of amenorrhoea), bleeding subsides within 48 hours and expectant management is an alternative to standard surgical curettage. Vaginal ultrasound helpful to confirm the diagnosis.

Missed abortion

- Occasionally, the fetus may die *in utero* but not be expelled. This is called a missed abortion.

Management

- If the uterus is less than 12 weeks, primary dilatation of the cervix and curettage or manual vacuum aspiration of the uterus is performed
- In those cases where the uterus is larger than 14 weeks, a medical induction using an abortifacient (misoprostol) should first be performed, followed by an evacuation after the abortion.

TERMINATION OF PREGNANCY ACT

According to the Act on Choice on Termination of Pregnancy of 1996, any pregnant woman, irrespective of age, can have a termination of pregnancy in the following circumstances or conditions:

- At her request during the first 12 weeks of pregnancy;
- From the 13th up to and including the 20th week of gestation if a medical practitioner, after consultation with the pregnant woman, is of the opinion that:
  - The continued pregnancy would pose a risk of injury to the woman's physical or mental health; or
  - There exists a substantial risk that the fetus would suffer from a severe physical or mental abnormality; or
  - The pregnancy resulted from rape or incest; or
  - The continued pregnancy would significantly affect the social or economic circumstances of the woman;
- After the 20th week of gestation if a medical practitioner, after consultation with another medical practitioner or a registered midwife who has completed the prescribed training course, is of the opinion that the continued pregnancy
  - Would endanger the woman's life; or
  - Would result in a severe malformation of the fetus; or
  - Would pose a risk of injury to the fetus.

The termination of pregnancy may only be performed by a medical practitioner, except for pregnancies under 13 weeks, which may also be carried out by trained registered midwives. No consent other than that of the pregnant woman is required.

INDUCED ABORTION

Methods of performing a termination of pregnancy
First trimester
- Cervical priming with vaginal misoprostol 2–4 hours prior to a suction curettage is the method of choice
- It must be noted that misoprostol is considered to be teratogenic and, once given it is mandatory to proceed with the termination of the pregnancy.

Second trimester
- In these cases, primary surgical curettage carries a relatively high risk
- Labour should first be induced and the fetus expelled before an evacuation is performed
- Usually prostaglandins are used for the induction; these are administered either orally or vaginally (misoprostol), or extra- or intra-amniotically (prostin F2α)
- Combinations of mifepristone, an antiprogesterone, in combination with misoprostol decrease the induction-abortion interval and make the procedure more predictable in outcome
- The usage of these drugs in the second trimester in patients with a previous

uterine scar carries a high risk of uterine rupture and should preferably be avoided. A safer alternative is mechanical dilatation using an intracervical balloon catheter.

Self-induced abortion
Self-induced abortion carries a high risk of maternal morbidity and mortality. The possibility of a self-induced abortion should be suspected in a patient with a complicated second trimester abortion.

COMPLICATIONS OF ABORTIONS

Septic abortion
Infection is a potential complication of any abortion, being especially common in unsafe abortions. The clinical entity of septic abortion results from infection and is one of the most serious complications.

Clinical picture
- Abortion is complicated by a fever (38 °C or higher)
- The site of sepsis located in the lower genital tract or uterine cavity
- Patients are often critically ill
- Septic abortion carries a 15 percent mortality risk.

Management
The strict management protocol used for critically ill pregnant women with complications of abortion includes the following principles:
- Stabilisation and resuscitation
- Antibiotics
- Evacuation or hysterectomy.

12 | Leiomyomata

T I Siebert, M Marivate

(See Chapter 16 in *Clinical Gynaecology*, 4th edition for more detailed information.)

A leiomyoma is a tumour of Müllerian duct origin, composed of smooth muscle interlaced with fibrous strands. They can be regarded as the most common form of neoplasm in the human body.

The different sites of leiomyomata are shown in Fig 12.1, below.

AETIOLOGY

The histogenesis of myomata has not been completely established.

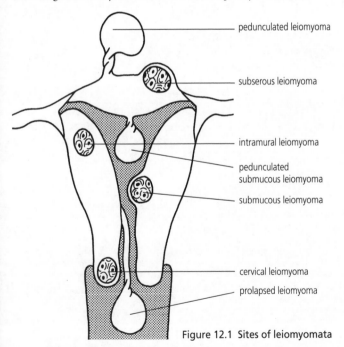

Figure 12.1 Sites of leiomyomata

pedunculated leiomyoma

subserous leiomyoma

intramural leiomyoma

pedunculated submucous leiomyoma

submucous leiomyoma

cervical leiomyoma

prolapsed leiomyoma

Types of degeneration

■ *Hyaline and cystic degeneration and calcification*
■ *Necrobiosis or red degeneration*
■ *Sarcomatous degeneration*: It is estimated that sarcomatous change will occur in 0.2–0.5 percent of leiomyomata. The rapid growth of a leiomyoma and the development of pain should alert the clinician to the fact that sarcomatous change may be taking place
■ *Metastasising uterine leiomyoma*: Metastasising leiomyomata are to all intents and purposes indistinguishable from benign leiomyomata, except that they spread to other pelvic organs, the omentum and the lungs.

COMPLICATIONS

Leiomyomata and pregnancy
First trimester

■ Red degeneration should be treated conservatively. It often settles down with no adverse effects on the pregnancy.
■ *Abruptio placentae*, on the other hand, must be treated actively and immediate delivery of the fetus is often necessary.
■ Submucosal and large intramural fibroids may cause recurrent miscarriage.

Second trimester

Necrobiosis and recurrent miscarriage may occur in the second trimester.

Third trimester

■ Premature rupture of membranes and premature labour may occur
■ *Abruptio placentae* is a late complication if the placenta implants on a fibroid
■ Infrequently, intrauterine growth retardation.

Intrapartum

■ Labour complications: include uterine inertia, fetal malpresentation and obstruction of the birth canal
■ During Caesarean section, large leiomyomata in the lower uterine segment may make a lower segment incision hazardous, thus indicating a classical upper segment approach.

Postpartum

■ Leiomyomata may interfere with contraction and retraction, resulting in postpartum haemorrhage.

Complications in nonpregnant women

■ Anaemia
■ Infection
■ Torsion
■ Ascites.

CLINICAL FEATURES

Leiomyomata occur in 5–25 percent of women over the age of 35 years. Leiomyomata are rare before puberty. Their peak incidence is between 35 and 45 years of age and they regress postmenopausally. Patients present with:

- Infertility
- Abdominal mass
- Pain
- Vaginal discharge
- Uterine inversion
- Pressure effects on bowel and urinary tract.

Ultrasonography may be helpful (and should always be carried out when the diagnosis of leiomyomata is entertained).

DIFFERENTIAL DIAGNOSIS

Genital tract

- Pregnancy (intra- and extrauterine)
- Ovarian tumours
- Inflammatory masses (including tuberculosis)
- Carcinoma of the endometrium
- Adenomyosis
- Endometriosis.

Urinary tract

- Bladder masses
- Kidney masses (pelvic kidney, horseshoe kidney).

TREATMENT

Surgery

Surgery should **be considered** under the following conditions:

- When the leiomyoma is larger than the size of the uterus, equivalent to a 14 weeks' gestation
- When the leiomyoma distorts the uterine cavity in a patient who wishes to have more children, provided that there are no other causes of infertility
- When the leiomyoma is situated in the lower part of the uterus, which may complicate labour
- When there is doubt about the nature of the leiomyoma
- In the presence of complications, for example severe menorrhagia, pain or pressure on neighbouring organs
- Sudden enlargement of a myoma
- The surgical procedures usually performed for leiomyomata are **abdominal hysterectomy, myomectomy, or hysteroscopic resection** of submucous myomas

- **Myomectomy** indicated in infertility cases
- **Hysteroscopy**, which in cases of infertility is combined with hysterosalpingography, may be indicated for the diagnosis of small submucous tumours.

Conservative treatment
It is generally agreed that no surgical intervention is necessary if leiomyomata are small, symptomless or discovered incidentally in women at the climacteric.

Medical treatment
See Chapter 16 of *Clinical Gynaecology*, 4th edition.

NOTES:

13 | Dysmenorrhoea

S Monokwane, T F Kruger

(See Chapter 17 in *Clinical Gynaecology*, 4th edition for more detailed information.)

DEFINITIONS

The word "dysmenorrhoea" is derived from Greek meaning "difficult menstrual flow" (or painful menstruation). Dysmenorrhoea is the most common gynaecological condition in adolescents, affecting 50–75 percent of menstruating females in the reproductive age group. It is severe in 10–15 percent.

There are two types of dysmenorrhoea:

- **Primary dysmenorrhoea** refers to painful menstrual cramps without underlying pathology
- **Secondary dysmenorrhoea** is painful menstrual cramps due to an underlying recognised pathology.

PRIMARY DYSMENORRHOEA

Clinical presentation

- Symptoms begin 2–3 hours before or within a few hours of the onset of menstrual flow
- Pain is in the form of spasmodic, labour-like cramps, which affect the lower abdomen and may radiate to the back and inner thighs
- Spasmodic pain, often with nausea and vomiting, is most intense on the first or second day of the menstrual flow.

Treatment

There are three approaches to the management of primary dysmenorrhoea. In all, the physician should give a careful explanation of the condition to the patient and emotional support where indicated.

- Pharmacological
- Non-pharmacological
- Surgical.

Pharmacological agents
Nonsteroidal anti-inflammatory drugs

NSAIDs relieve primary dysmenorrhoea by inhibiting endometrial prostaglandin production and release. They also have a direct analgesic effect centrally. They are effective in 80–90 percent of cases.

Carboxylic acids are the first choice, prescribed at the onset of menstruation, and they include propionic acids:

- Ibuprofen 400–800 mg po 6-hourly
- Naproxen 250–500 mg po 6-hourly.

Oral contraceptives

The combined oral contraceptive pill inhibits ovulation and leads to thinning of the endometrium. This will result in lower levels of menstrual fluid volume with prostaglandins and thus relief of dysmenorrhoea in up to 90 percent of women.

Other supplements

- Vitamin B6 has proved to be more effective than a placebo in reducing menstrual pain.
- Magnesium supplements are also helpful.

Non-pharmacological agents

- Transcutaneous Electrical Nerve stimulation (TENS)
- Acupuncture
- Hot water bottle.

Surgical treatment
Surgical ablation

The use of uterosacral nerve ablation (LUNA) and presacral neurectomy for primary dysmenorrhoea is reserved for severe non-responders to medical therapy.

SECONDARY DYSMENORRHOEA

The menstrual pain of secondary dysmenorrhoea occurs with or is secondary to an underlying pelvic pathology. The onset is usually more than two years following menarche.

Possible causes of secondary dysmenorrhoea
Extrauterine

- Endometriosis
- Tumours or fibroids
- Pelvic infection or PID
- Pelvic congestion syndrome
- Adhesions
- Psychogenic factors
- Müllerian tract anomalies
- Intramural myomas
- Adenomyosis.

Intrauterine
- Myomas
- Polyps
- IUCD
- Cervical stenosis or lesions
- Infection.

Non-gynaecological
- GIT
- Urinary infection
- Orthopaedic disorder.

14 | Pelvic pain

D R Hall

(See Chapter 18 in *Clinical Gynaecology*, 4th edition for more detailed information.)

HISTORY

The history is central to the diagnosis

- Time of onset and nature of the pain
- Symptoms from other organs, for example bowel, bladder, muscles, skeleton
- Gynaecological history
- Sexual history including superficial or deep dyspareunia and infections
- Family history
- Social history including relationship problems, stress and sexual abuse.

EXAMINATION

- Note the woman's general mood and make observations
- During the abdominal examination, look for distension, masses, pain and areas of tenderness
- Pain may be accompanied by guarding or rebound tenderness. Auscultation would be performed if ileus were suspected
- Perform a vaginal and rectal examination
- Inspection may reveal bleeding or an abnormal discharge suggestive of infection
- Take a cervical smear as appropriate
- The bimanual examination may reveal an enlarged uterus or adnexa as, for example, with fibroids (leiomyomata) or an ovarian cyst
- Cervical excitation tenderness may be present, indicating pelvic peritoneal irritation by a bleeding ectopic pregnancy or infection
- Tenderness of the pelvic organs during bimanual examination may also be a sign of infection or distortion, for example adhesions or stretching of the visceral peritoneum over an ovarian cyst.

IMPORTANT CAUSES OF ACUTE PELVIC PAIN

- **Pregnancy-associated pain**: miscarriage, ectopic pregnancy
- **Pain of gynaecological origin**: dysmenorrhoea, salpingitis/pelvic inflammatory disease, endometriosis, red degeneration of a leiomyoma, adnexal cyst/tumour with bleeding, torsion or rupture
- **Pain of nongynaecological origin**: urological, gastroenterological and musculoskeletal causes

- **Urological causes:** acute urethritis, urethral diverticulum, acute cystitis, radiation cystitis, renal calculus, pyelonephritis
- **Gastroenterological causes:** appendicitis, diverticulitis, bowel obstruction
- **Musculoskeletal causes:** disc lesion.

CHRONIC PELVIC PAIN (CPP)

Definition: intermittent or constant pain in the lower abdomen or pelvis of at least six months' duration, not occurring exclusively with menstruation or intercourse and not associated with pregnancy.

Key points

Pelvic pain is not a diagnosis but rather a symptom with a number of contributory factors.

- Social, physical and psychological factors influence the perception of pain
- CPP is best managed within a multidisciplinary setting
- In up to 50 percent of investigated cases no clear organic pathology is found
- In such cases the doctor–patient relationship should be nonjudgemental, involve the patient's concerns and establish realistic expectations.

Diagnosis

- History and examination followed by selected special investigations
- Non-invasive imaging modalities such as ultrasound
- Diagnostic laparoscopy should be regarded as a second line investigation.

IMPORTANT CAUSES OF CHRONIC PELVIC PAIN

- Endometriosis
- Adenomyosis
- Adhesions
- Pelvic inflammatory disease
- Ovarian cysts and leiomyomata
- Pelvic venous congestion
- Gastrointestinal causes
- Musculoskeletal causes
- Nerve entrapment in scar tissue
- Urological causes
- Psychosocial causes.

KEY POINTS

- A thorough history including psychosocial factors is important
- Always consider other organ systems
- A complete gynaecological examination must be performed
- Perform only indicated special investigations. Pelvic ultrasound and laparoscopy are useful tests

- When no gynaecological cause is found for the pain, discuss this openly with the woman without implying that there is "nothing wrong". Further unnecessary investigations and even operations should be avoided in an attempt to "buy time". A caring multidisciplinary approach is important
- Devise strategies to relieve the physical and psychosocial distress of CPP.

15 | Abnormal uterine bleeding

J S Bagratee

(See Chapter 19 in *Clinical Gynaecology*, 4th edition for more detailed information.)

DEFINITIONS

- **Menorrhagia** means excessive menstrual bleeding.
- **Metrorrhagia** means irregular bleeding at any time between menstrual periods.
- **Polymenorrhoea** refers to bleeding episodes that occur over less than 21 days.
- **Oligomenorrhoea** means scanty menstruation or long menstrual cycles over 35 days.
- **Normal bleeding** lasts 2 to 5 days every 23 to 33 days. However cycles must be regular, for example someone presenting with a 23 day cycle (the cycle should not vary with more than 1 or 2 days). A variation of for example 23 to 31 days or 33 days is not normal, therefore irregular.
- **Objective menorrhagia** is defined as a blood loss of greater than 80 ml per cycle.

CAUSES OF ABNORMAL UTERINE BLEEDING

- **Dysfunctional uterine bleeding**
- **Abnormal pregnancy states**
  - Miscarriage
  - Ectopic pregnancy
  - Gestational trophoblastic disease
- **Blood dyscrasias**
  - Thrombocytopenia
  - Von Willebrand's disease
  - Leukaemia
- **Genital tract pathology**
  - Congenital uterine abnormalities
  - Trauma
  - Infection
  - Endometriosis and adenomyosis
  - Benign neoplasms, for example polyps, fibroids, hyperplasias
  - Malignant neoplasms, for example carcinomas, sarcomas, hormone-producing tumours
- **Iatrogenic**
  - Hormonal contraceptives

- Hormone replacement therapy
- Intrauterine contraceptive device
- Anticoagulant therapy
- Haemodialysis
- **Endocrine causes**
  - Hypothyroidism
  - Adrenal disorders
- **Systemic disorders**
  - Hepatic disease
  - Renal disease
  - Obesity
- **Psychological disorders**.

MANAGEMENT OF ABNORMAL UTERINE BLEEDING/ MENORRHAGIA

- Information and reassurance
- Detailed menstrual calendar
- Haematinics
- Treatment of psychological and/or emotional problems
- Tranexamic acid 1 g 6-hourly
- Nonsteroidal anti-inflammatory drugs (NSAIDs) reduce prostaglandin synthesis by inhibiting the cyclo-oxygenase enzyme
- Combined oral contraceptive pills are useful in reducing menstrual bleeding
- Levonorgestrel intrauterine system
- Endometrial ablation
- Hysterectomy if:
  - The woman has completed her family and is over 45 years of age
  - Medical treatment has failed
  - There are premalignant conditions of the cervix and/or endometrium
  - Endometrial ablation has failed.

MANAGEMENT OF THE ACUTE BLEEDING EPISODE

- Combination oral contraceptive pill is effective if the bleeding is not severe
- Norethisterone 10–30 mg per day is administered for seven to ten days
- 25 mg conjugated equine oestrogen IV if bleeding is due to an atrophic endometrium
- Oral conjugated equine oestrogen in the dose of 2.5 mg three times a day is also recommended (Premarin®)
- Tranexamic acid (cyclokapron acetate) parenterally in a dose of 1.5 g.

16 | Antibiotic therapy and genital tract infection

D J Botha, P Roos

(See Chapter 11: "Antibiotic therapy in gynaecology" and Chapter 10: "Infections of the genital tract", in *Clinical Gynaecology*, 4th edition, for more detailed information.)

ANTIBIOTICS IN PREGNANCY

Some antibiotics used in gynaecological practice are contra-indicated in pregnancy. It is therefore essential that the possibility of pregnancy be considered whenever these drugs are prescribed.

FUNDAMENTAL PRINCIPLES OF SURGICAL PROPHYLAXIS

- The antibiotic must be in the tissue before the bacteria are introduced, that is antibiotic must be given intravenously shortly before surgery to ensure high blood/tissue levels. If metronidazole is administered as a rectal suppository, it should be given 2–4 hours preoperatively. A single preoperative dose has the same efficacy as multiple doses and the current recommendation is to administer a second dose only if the operation lasts for longer than 2–3 hours.
- Antibiotics must be of low toxicity.
- There is no data to support more than a single dose. Further doses generally constitute treatment.
- The chosen antibiotic must be active against the most common expected pathogens.
- High-risk patients, for example patients with jaundice or diabetes, or patients undergoing any procedures to insert prosthetic devices, generally warrant antibiotic prophylaxis.
- There are no convincing statistical differences in efficacy between the first-, second- or third-generation cephalosporins, therefore a first-generation cephalosporin must be the preferred option.

RECOMMENDATIONS ON ANTIBIOTIC PROPHYLAXIS

Prophylactic antibiotics ought not to replace good operative standards. These include:

Preoperatively
- Cleaning of operative site
- Washing of hands
- Wearing of sterile gowns and gloves
- Sterilising of instruments.

Intraoperatively
- Careful surgical technique with gentle handling of tissue
- Good haemostasis
- Avoiding unnecessary tissue necrosis by keeping the size of pedicles to a minimum
- Reducing foreign body reaction by using fine, nonreactive suture material.

Postoperatively
- Washing of hands
- Isolation of infected patients
- Proper disposal of all infected material.

The principle is that antibiotic prophylaxis should be to the benefit of the receiving patient but should not constitute a danger for others in the same environment.

INTRAVENOUS ANTIBIOTIC THERAPY FOR POSTOPERATIVE INFECTIONS

Localised infection with minimal systemic findings
- **Cefoxitin** (Mefoxin®), 2 g every 6 hours or
- **Ceftriaxone** (Rocephin®), 2 g followed by 1g every 24 hours

Extensive infection with moderate to severe systemic findings
- **Clindamycin** (Dalacin C®), 900 mg IV every 8 hours plus
- **Gentamycin** (Garamycin®), given as a single daily dose of 5 mg/kg IV
- **Ampicillin, penicillin** or **vancomycin** (Vancocin CP®) may be added to cover enterococci.

If vancomycin-resistant enterococci are proved to be the cause of a serious infection, treat with:
- **Imipenem/cilastatin** (Tienam®), 500 mg to 1 000 mg IV every 6 hours or
- **Levofloxacin** (Tavanic®) 500 mg IV every 24 hours plus
- **Metronidazole** 500 mg IV every 8 hours can be used.

SEXUAL ASSAULT AND STD PROPHYLAXIS

Trichomoniasis, bacterial vaginosis (BV), gonorrhoea and chlamydial infection are the most frequently diagnosed infections among women who have been sexually assaulted.

The following prophylactic regimen is suggested as preventive therapy:
- Postexposure hepatitis B vaccination, without HBIG, should adequately protect against HBV infection. Hepatitis B vaccination should be administered to sexual assault victims at the time of the initial examination if they have not been previously vaccinated. Follow-up doses of vaccine should be administered 1–2 and 4–6 months after the first dose.
- An empiric antimicrobial regimen for chlamydia, gonorrhoea, trichomonas and BV.

- Emergency contraception should be offered if the assault could result in pregnancy in the survivor.
- Antiretroviral therapy as per institutional guidelines.

Table 16.1 Recommended prophylactic regimens after sexual assault

Ceftriaxone (Rocephin®) 125 mg IM in a single dose PLUS
Metronidazole (Flagyl®) 2 g orally in a single dose PLUS

Azithromycin (Zithromax®) 1 g orally in a single dose OR
Doxycycline (Cyclidox®) 100 mg orally twice a day for 7 days.

GYNAECOLOGICAL INFECTIONS AND ORGANISM-SPECIFIC TREATMENT

Table 16.2 Gynaecological infections and organism specific treatment

Organism and/ or illness type	Drug of choice	Adult dose	Alternative
Acute urethritis (males)	**Ceftriaxone** (Rocephin®) OR **Ciprofloxacin*** (Ciprobay®)	250 mg IM 500 mg PO stat	
Vaginal trichomoniasis	**Metronidazole** (Flagyl®)	400 mg PO 12 hourly X 7 days OR single dose 2 g orally	Tinidazole (Fasigyn 500®) 2 g PO as a single dose
Vaginal candidiasis			
Non-pregnant	**Clotrimazole** (Canesten®)	500 mg vaginal tab once OR 2 X 100 mg vaginal tab nocte X 3 nights OR vaginal (1 percent) cream nocte X 6 nights	Miconazole (Gyno-Daktarin®) OR Tioconazole (Gyno-Trosyd®) OR Econazole (Gyno-Pevaryl®)
	OR		
	Fluconazole (Diflucan®)	150 mg PO as a single dose	Itraconazole (Sporanox®) 200 mg 12 hourly x 2 doses

*Where quinolone resistance has been reported, cephalosporin therapy should be regarded as treatment choice.

GENITAL TRACT INFECTIONS WITH DISCHARGE

Vaginal candida
- Thick white to green discharge with itching, burning and erythema. Associated with antibiotic therapy, diabetes mellitus, immune deficiency states, pregnancy and the contraceptive pill
- Diagnosis is made on clinical appearance and microscopy using a potassium hydroxide wet preparation showing thread like pseudohyphae

Bacterial vaginosis
- White, grey discharge with odour and little or no irritation or erythema
- Diagnosis made with potassium hydroxide "whiff test" and the presence of clue cells on microscopy.

Trichomonas
- Yellow green frothy discharge with burning and odour, erythema particularly of the upper vagina and cervix
- Diagnosis wet preparation with sodium chloride showing mobile protozoa under microscopy.

Mixed bacterial infection
- Yellow brown malodorous discharge associated with neoplasms, trauma, foreign bodies, pelvic inflammatory disease and retained products of conception
- Diagnosis made on clinical appearance and culture of specific bacteria
- Treatment – appropriate antibiotics and management of the underlying cause.

Chlamydia
- Non specific vaginal discharge, sometimes asymptomatic, occasionally causing discomfort with or without erythema
- Diagnosis using polymerase chain reaction test on urine or cervical swabs.

INFECTIONS WITH A VISIBLE LESION

Human papillomavirus (HPV)
- Typical genital and peri-anal warts varying from pinpoint size to enormous
- Diagnosis on clinical appearance and biopsy
- Treatment: smaller warts may be treated with local preparation such as podophylox, imiquimod or a saturated solution of Trichloric acid. Genital warts may also be surgically removed or treated with electro-cautery, laser therapy or cryotherapy.

Herpes genitalis
- Clinical history and examination is usually diagnostic. There is initially burning, itching or discomfort on a localised area of skin on the genital

area. This is followed by red papules which become vesicles which rupture leaving painful ulceration. This clinical course is about 4–5 days.
■ Diagnosis by means of laboratory investigations is often expensive and serology useful primarily in the first infection. Should diagnosis be difficult you should discuss the diagnostic measures such as viral cultures and electro-microscopy with your local laboratory.

Primary syphilis
■ Typical lesion of primary syphilis is the chancre occurring either on the external genitalia or hidden within the vagina and cervix. The chancre changes from a macular papular lesion to an ulcer with a clean border and is usually painless, as are the regional lymph nodes associated with it.

Secondary syphilis
■ Condylomata lata are typically flat wart like growths differing from papillomavirus, which are pointed and thicker
■ Diagnosis of syphilis is primarily done by serology although the Treponema Pallidum can sometimes be seen on dark ground microscopy in the early stages when the serology has not yet become positive.

Haemophilus ducreyi
■ Chancroid is the clinical manifestation on the genital area. Papules are followed by pustules which then break down leaving ulceration. The ulceration has a ragged edge and tends to have a purulent base. Unlike syphilis the associated lymph nodes become very painful and associated with abscess formation.
■ Diagnosis is usually made on a clinical basis, but culture of purulent material can prove useful.

Lymphogranuloma venereum
■ This starts with a painless papule or blister followed in a period of up to 6 weeks by painful inguinal and femoral lymph nodes. They may also be associated with systemic symptoms. The lymph nodes can form abscesses which subsequently break down with sinus formation.

Calymmatobacterium granulomatis (granuloma inguinale)
■ This condition occurs more commonly in the tropics starting with small painless papules. These eventually break down to full granulomatous ulcers which eventually result in scarring. Lymph node involvement is rare.
■ Diagnosis is made on histology and staining of the organisms.

NOTES:

17 | Premenstrual tension

H M Sebitloane

(See Chapter 20 in *Clinical Gynaecology*, 4th edition for more detailed information.)

DEFINITIONS

Premenstrual tension is a cluster of predictable physical, psychological and behavioural symptoms which recur regularly and occur specifically during the luteal phase of the menstrual cycle, resolving with the onset of or during menstruation. The more severe form which presents predominantly with affective symptoms is referred to as premenstrual dysphoric disorder (PMDD), and requires more stringent diagnostic criteria.

EPIDEMIOLOGY

Up to 90 percent of menstruating women experience at least one mild symptom before their menses without disruption in their daily activities. Of these, about 20–40 percent of women have symptoms that are severe enough to impair daily functioning and are labelled PMS. The two ends of the spectrum are represented by 5 percent of women who are completely free of symptoms and about 2–6 percent of women with PMDD.

DIAGNOSIS

For diagnosis of PMS/PMDD, symptoms must be shown not only to be related to the luteal phase of the menstrual cycle, but also be absent during the period from the end of menstruation and ovulation. Additionally, the symptoms must:

- Be documented over several menstrual cycles (at least 2 consecutive cycles, prospectively recorded)
- Not be explained by other physical or psychological conditions
- Cause impairment and interfere with work, social activities and/or relationships.

The patients should manifest any of the symptoms as listed in Table 17.1. For PMS, there should be at least one of the affective and one of the somatic symptoms, however, other authorities will accept at least one symptom of sufficient severity to lead to disruption of daily activities.

On the other hand, stringent criteria are needed for the diagnosis of PMDD, which is thought to be a more severe and debilitating condition. Out of the 11 symptoms listed in the DSM-IV, at least 5 are needed, one of which should primarily be a mood disorder for the positive diagnosis of PMDD.

TREATMENT

For women with mild to moderate symptoms, conservative management is advisable, including emotional support, supplements and exercise. Treatment options are summarised in Figure 17.1. About 30 percent of PMS patients have their symptoms reduced sufficiently with the use of first-line conservative measures.

Conservative management of PMS

- Education, support, stress reduction and exercise: Management should also include the regulation and improvement of sleep habits
- Dietary modification: Although widely recommended, dietary modification has never been evaluated in a controlled, scientific manner
- Nutritional supplements:
  - Calcium supplementation at a dosage of 1 000 mg per day significantly reduces both the physical and emotional symptoms of PMS
  - Magnesium 360 mg per day significantly reduces water retention and the negative effect associated with PMS
  - It is also beneficial to use a nutritional supplement consisting of evening primrose oil (Efamol G®).

Medical Management

Depending on the severity of symptoms, patients with severe disease will require treatment targeted at symptoms, whilst the diagnosis is still being established. These may include bromocriptine for breast tenderness or anxiolytics for emotional stability. Once diagnosis is made, the most effective therapies are those shown to inhibit ovulation, as well as mood stabilisers such as selective serotonin reuptake inhibitors. Medical management can be targeted at relieving symptoms, or addressing possible causative factors.

Physical symptoms

As a general rule, physical symptoms are treated first, since improvement in emotional symptoms frequently accompanies improvement in physical symptoms.

- Water-retention symptoms: spironolactone 25 mg up to four times a day
- Mastalgia may be treated with diuretic therapy or with bromocriptine 2.5 mg nightly, increasing to 2.5 mg twice daily from day 10 of the cycle
- Prostaglandins mediate many of the pain-related symptoms of PMS. Mefenamic acid should be prescribed at a dosage of 500 mg three times daily.

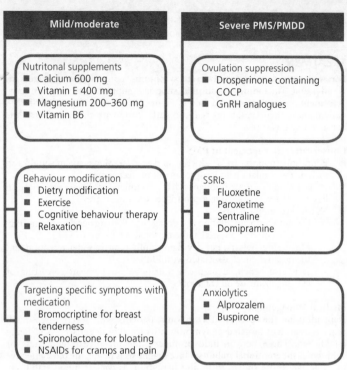

Mild/moderate	Severe PMS/PMDD
Nutritonal supplements ■ Calcium 600 mg ■ Vitamin E 400 mg ■ Magnesium 200–360 mg ■ Vitamin B6	Ovulation suppression ■ Drosperinone containing COCP ■ GnRH analogues
Behaviour modification ■ Dietry modification ■ Exercise ■ Cognitive behaviour therapy ■ Relaxation	SSRIs ■ Fluoxetine ■ Paroxetime ■ Sentraline ■ Domipramine
Targeting specific symptoms with medication ■ Bromocriptine for breast tenderness ■ Spironolactone for bloating ■ NSAIDs for cramps and pain	Anxiolytics ■ Alprozalem ■ Buspirone

Figure 17.1 Management algorithm for management of PMS/PMDD.

Ovulation suppression
■ Drospirenone: Drospirenone is a progestin that is an analogue of spironolactone and exhibits antiandrogenic and anti-mineralocorticoid activity. It is thus effective in the treatment of PMS and is currently the treatment of choice. Yasmin® and especially its newer preparation YAZ® (containing 20µg rather than 30µg, and is administered for 24 days of active pills – 24/4 rather than 21/7) are now considered as **first line treatment** of women with PMS/PMDD and requiring contraception. YAZ®, the 24/4 preparation is thought to be more effective by providing more stable hormonal levels and reducing adverse symptoms that can occur during withdrawal bleeding, and has been approved by the FDA in the United States since 2006 for treatment of PMS/PMDD.
■ GnRH agonists.

Emotional symptoms

It is currently recognised that the three major emotional PMS problems – namely irritability, affect lability and depressed mood – are related to brain responsiveness to sex steroids.

- Fluoxetine (Prozac®) is an effective and well-tolerated treatment of severe PMS
- Alprazolam (Xanor®) is a triazolobenzodiazepine with anxiolytic, antidepressant and smooth-muscle relaxant properties.

Table 17.1 Criteria for premenstrual dysphoric disorder adapted from the DSM–IV–TR

A. In most menstrual cycles during the past year, five (or more) of the following symptoms were present for most of the time during the last week of the luteal phase, began to remit within a few days after the onset of the follicular phase, and were absent in the week after menses, with at least one of the symptoms being 1, 2, 3, or 4:
1. Markedly depressed mood, feelings of hopelessness, or self-deprecating thoughts.
2. Marked anxiety, tension, feelings of being "keyed up," or "on edge."
3. Marked affective lability (e.g., feeling suddenly sad or tearful, or increased sensitivity to rejection).
4. Persistent and marked anger or irritability or increased interpersonal conflicts.
5. Decreased interest in usual activities (e.g., work, school, friends, hobbies).
6. Subjective sense of difficulty in concentrating.
7. Lethargy, easy fatigability, or marked lack of energy.
8. Marked change in appetite, overeating, or specific food cravings.
9. Hypersomnia or insomnia.
10. Subjective sense of being overwhelmed or out of control.
11. Physical symptoms, such as breast tenderness or swelling, headaches, joint or muscle pain, a sensation of "bloating," weight gain.
B. The disturbance markedly interferes with work or school or with usual social activities and relationships with others.
C. The disturbance is not merely an exacerbation of the symptoms of another disorder.
D. Criteria A, B, and C must be confirmed by prospective daily rating during at least two consecutive symptomatic cycles.

NOTES:

18 | Amenorrhoea, oligomenorrhoea, galactorrhoea

Z M van der Spuy

(See Chapter 25 in *Clinical Gynaecology*, 4th edition for more detailed information.)

The absence of menstruation occurs as a physiological event during pregnancy and lactation, before normal menarche, and after the menopause. In other circumstances, amenorrhoea warrants investigation since it may be indicative of significant underlying pathology.

The main causes of amenorrhoea are listed in Table 18.1 below.

Table 18.1 Aetiology of amenorrhoea

1. **Physiological**
   (i) Pregnancy
   (ii) Lactation

2. **CNS and hypothalamus**
   (i) Psycho-neuroendocrinological factors:
   - Stress
   - Pseudocyesis (phantom pregnancy)
   - Undernutrition
     - anorexia nervosa
     - "simple" weight loss
     - exercise
   (ii) GnRH deficiency (Kallmann's syndrome)
   (iii) Compression or destruction of hypothalamus by CNS tumours – usually extrasellar masses, e.g. craniopharyngioma, metastases.

3. **Pituitary gland**
   (i) Hyperprolactinaemic states:
   - Pituitary tumour
   - Pharmacological causes
   - Intracranial lesion, e.g. craniopharyngioma
   - Physiological causes
   - Peripheral causes, e.g. hypothyroidism
   (ii) Cellular and anatomic defects causing hypopituitarism:
   - Isolated gonadotropin deficiency
   - Non-neoplastic intracellular masses, e.g. tuberculosis, sarcoidosis
   - Empty-sella syndrome
   - Irradiation

      (iii) Other pituitary causes:
- Functional adenomas, e.g. Cushing's syndrome, acromegaly
- Non-functioning adenomas

      (iv) Disruption of hypothalamic-pituitary connections:
- Stalk lesions
  - trauma
  - tumour
- Ischaemia and infarction (Sheehan's syndrome).

4. Gonadal causes
  (i) Primary ovarian failure:
- Dysgenesis
- Damage, e.g. surgery, irradiation
- Premature menopause
- Autoantibodies

  (ii) Gonadal dysfunction:
- Polycystic ovary syndrome
- Functional ovarian tumours.

5. End-organ defects
  (i) Congenital abnormalities:
- Müllerian agenesis (Mayer-Rokitansky-Küster-Hauser syndrome)
- Müllerian anomalies
- Disorders of sexual differential (DSD)
  - deficient testosterone synthesis
  - 5α-reductase deficiency
  - androgen insensitivity
  - fetal and postnatal androgen excess

  (ii) Acquired abnormalities:
- Obliteration or obstruction of uterine cavity or cervix.

6. Thyroid gland
- Hypothyroidism
- Hyperthyroidism.

7. Adrenal gland
- Congenital adrenal hyperplasia
- Cushing's syndrome
- Addison's syndrome.

8. Metabolic condition
- Vegan diet
- Diabetes mellitus
- Liver disease.

9. Medication
- Impacts at many levels of the hypothalamic pituitary ovarian (HPO) axis and outflow tract.

Any woman complaining of amenorrhoea who fulfils the following criteria warrants investigation:

- 14 years of age with no secondary sexual characteristics (delayed puberty)
- 16 years of age with normal growth and development of secondary sexual characteristics (delayed menarche)
- Amenorrhoea for three to six months (post-menarche) (opinions vary on the duration)
- Signs of hyperandrogenism regardless of the duration of menstrual dysfunction
- Dysmorphic features
- Signs of any endocrinopathy.

INVESTIGATIONS AND MANAGEMENT

In summary, a practical approach to the woman with amenorrhoea may be planned as follows.

First visit

- Clinical assessment
- Exclude pregnancy
- Special investigations:
  - progestogen withdrawal
  - prolactin
  - FSH, LH, TSH
  - androgens, if indicated
- Chromosome analysis if:
  - short stature (<1.52 m)
  - suspected abnormality
  - primary amenorrhoea
- Pelvic ultrasonography.

Follow-up visit

Correlate results and reassess for further investigations.

- FSH elevated – consider gonadal failure
- LH elevated, FSH normal – consider PCOS, assess androgen status, review ultrasonography
- Prolactin elevated – perform radiology of pituitary gland
- Androgens elevated:
  - DHEAS raised – full adrenal assessment;
  - testosterone raised – consider ovarian origin
- PCO on ultrasonographic examination – further investigations.

19 | An alternative approach to make a diagnosis in patients with amenorrhoea

T F Kruger

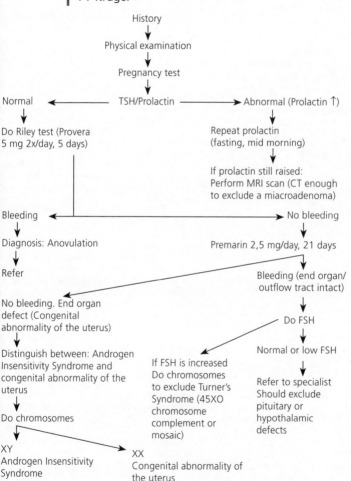

Figure 19.1 An alternative approach to make a diagnosis in patients with amenorrhoea.

20 | Hyperandrogenism

Z M van der Spuy

(See Chapter 26 in *Clinical Gynaecology*, 4th edition for more detailed information.)

The clinical presentation of hyperandrogenism varies considerably and androgen excess may be a marker of serious underlying pathology.

DEFINITIONS

- **Hyperandrogenism.** The condition of increased androgen production or action.
- **Hirsutism.** The growth of terminal hair in amounts that is socially undesirable. Characteristically, follicles on the face, upper lip, breasts, lower abdomen and upper thighs are induced to grow in a male pattern.
- **Acne vulgaris.** This is not an endocrine disease but it is hormonally influenced. Androgens increase the rate of mitosis and epithelial proliferation of the sebaceous gland acini and cause enhanced sebum production. Both acne vulgaris and a greasy skin may therefore be manifestations of hyperandrogenism.
- **Virilisation.** This is the development of male secondary sexual characteristics in a woman. These may include severe hirsutism associated with defeminisation, clitoromegaly, deepening of the voice and sometimes temporal balding. Muscle bulk increases and the body habitus is altered. Plasma androgen levels may approach those of the male range. Virilisation is virtually always indicative of organic disease.
- **Hypertrichosis.** This is a general increase in terminal hair density with the occasional appearance of terminal hair in abnormal sites. This is not an androgen-dependent condition and there are multiple causes, including porphyria, head injury and drugs such as phenytoin and diazoxide.

ANDROGENS IN WOMEN

Testosterone, androstenedione and dehydroepiandrosterone (DHEA) are the three main naturally occurring androgens. Androstenedione and DHEA exert their androgenic influence after peripheral conversion to testosterone (which is biologically the most important androgen) in tissue such as fat, skin, muscle and liver. Testosterone in turn is converted to the very potent androgen, DHT, by the enzyme 5α-reductase and this step is necessary in many tissues before expression of androgenicity.

CLINICAL ASSESSMENT

The hyperandrogenised woman may present with a variety of clinical complaints. The most common presentation is an unacceptable increase in hair. The distribution and severity of the hirsutism may vary considerably from patient to patient. The patient may also complain of acne, which often has proven resistant to simple therapy. Sometimes she presents with virilisation and this requires urgent investigation since the hyperandrogenaemia may be caused by a tumour. Menstrual abnormalities or infertility may be the main complaint, with the patient admitting to hirsutism or virilisation only on closer questioning. A careful history and examination is essential.

SPECIAL INVESTIGATIONS

These aim at establishing the origin and cause of the hyperandrogenism. They may include:

- Serum testosterone
- SHBG – use this to calculate the free androgen index: (testosterone × 100) ÷ SHBG
- DHEAS: mainly adrenal in origin
- FSH and LH – of limited value
- 17α hydroxyprogesterone to exclude CAH
- Tests to exclude Cushing's syndrome
- Thyroid function tests
- Ultrasonography of the ovaries
- Specialised radiology.

SUMMARY

In summary, a practical approach to this clinical problem involves at least the following:

- Some estimation of testosterone
- DHEAS and 17α-OH progesterone to exclude adrenal disease
- If the FSH : LH ratio is abnormal and/or testosterone levels elevated, ultrasonography of the ovaries may confirm the diagnosis of PCOS or localise an ovarian tumour
- If DHEAS and 17α-OHP are abnormal, further testing is essential to exclude adrenal pathology
- If all investigations are normal, a presumed increase in end-organ sensitivity can be postulated.

INDICATIONS FOR EXTREMELY URGENT INVESTIGATION OF HYPERANDROGENISM INCLUDE:

- Rapid progression of hyperandrogenism – suspect a tumour
- Very high testosterone levels – suspect a tumour
- Failure of therapy – reconsider diagnosis.

21 | Paediatric gynaecology

C M C Dehaeck

(See Chapter 56 in *Clinical Gynaecology* 4th edition, for more detailed information.)

Paediatric gynaecology is a comprehensive term used for gynaecological conditions that range from the newborn to the young female child to commencement of normal puberty.

THE EXAMINATION

- A gynaecological examination should be done with the parent or caretaker present
- Indications are pathological conditions, sexual abuse suspicion or reassurance about abnormality
- Detailed history is necessary
- External genitalia are examined in the rooms
- General anaesthetic may sometimes be necessary, but never conscious sedation
- Position supine, left lateral, knee chest or sitting on a lap
- Visualisation in general
- Open the labia to have a closer look, and pull the labia majora gently towards you to inspect the hymen
- Good lighting, nasal speculum, a vaginoscope, hysteroscope or cystoscope is needed in theatre.

PHYSIOLOGICAL CHANGES

Can be seen in the newborn secondary to oestrogen circulation from the mother:
- Nipple discharge
- Slight breast enlargement
- Clear vaginal discharge
- Some withdrawal bleeding.

The examining doctor needs to have knowledge of the normal anatomy and physiology.

PATHOLOGICAL CONDITIONS

Congenital abnormalities

1. Hypertrophy of the clitoris
- Relative enlargement can be normal in the female infant
- Intersex conditions (for example androgen-producing tumour)
- Intake of androgen by the mother
- Surgery should be delayed until after puberty.

2. Hypertrophy of the labia minora
- May need surgery if worrisome after puberty.

3. Imperforate hymen
- May present as hydrocolpos in the infant and heamatocolpos, after menarche
- Treatment is incision of the hymen under general anaesthetic.

4. Transverse vaginal septum
- This can be low or high, and surgical excision is necessary because it also presents with haematocolpos or haematometria.

5. Ectopic ureter
- A rare condition which causes continuous wetting
- Ureter needs to be transplanted into bladder.

6. Congenital absence of the vagina and/or blind ending vagina
- Discussed in Chapter 23 of *Clinical Gynaecology*, 4th edition.

7. Intersex
- Discussed in Chapter 23 of *Clinical Gynaecology*, 4th edition.

Labial adhesions
- Common condition: aetiology is unknown
- Treatment necessary if it causes discomfort or accumulation of urine behind the adhesion
- Treatment: 10–14 days of oestrogen cream application
- Rarely is it necessary to do a separation in theatre.

Infections
Non specific vulvovaginitis
Aetiology
- Lack of protective acid environment
- Lack of vulvar fat pads
- Proximity of anus to the opening of the vagina
- Lack of hygiene
- Foreign material

- Obesity
- Impaired immunity
- Dominant bacteria usually faecal in origin
- Can be transferred from other infections.

Treatment
Oestrogen for two weeks or specific antibiotics if culture of high vaginal swab indicates a specific bacterium.

Specific vulvovaginitis
Candida albicans infections:
Rare, premenarchal except in the use of long-term antibiotics or diabetes mellitus. Treatment: antifungals.

Threadworms
Treatment: deworming.

Sexually transmitted diseases
- Trichomonas
- *Neisseria gonorrhoeae*
- Genital herpes
- Chlamydial infections.

These need to be treated appropriately as in the adult.

Human immunodeficiency virus (HIV) should be considered in all sexually abused children, and children presenting with sexually transmitted diseases. Counselling is of utmost importance in these cases.

Vaginal bleeding
This usually indicates pathology and needs an examination under anaesthetic to exclude:
- Infection
- Prolapse of the urethral mucosa
- Foreign material
- Sexual abuse or trauma
- Precocious menarche
- Rare tumours of the vagina and cervix.

A high vaginal swab needs to be taken and detailed notes kept.

DERMATOLOGICAL CONDITIONS OF THE VULVA
Lichen sclerosus et atrophicus
- A white lesion of the vulva causing pruritus

- Can present with subcutaneous bleeds
- If necessary a biopsy needs to be taken for diagnosis, and the treatment is corticosteroid cream.

Dermatitis
- Can be an allergic reaction, and allergic irritation
- Eczema
- Psoriasis.

Precocious puberty
- This is the appearance of any element in pubertal development before the age of 8
- Can be telarche, adenarche or menarche (see Chapter 24 of *Clinical Gynaecology*, 4th edition).

GYNAECOLOGICAL TUMOURS

These are rare:
- Ovarian cyst and neoplasms
- Polyps of the vagina
- Sarcoma botryoides
- Clear cell adenocarcinoma of the vagina.

TRAUMA

- This can be caused by foreign objects or during sexual abuse
- If this has led to bleeding an examination under general anaesthetic is indicated
- If the posterior fornix has been penetrated a laparotomy or laparoscopy is needed to exclude bowel damage.

SUMMARY

The examination of a young female child needs to be conducted keeping the United Nations (UN) convention of the "Rights of the child" in mind.

22 | Infertility

T F Kruger, J P van der Merwe

(See Chapter 27: "Female infertility" and Chapter 28: "Male infertility" in *Clinical Gynaecology*, 4th edition for more detailed information.)

Infertility is a complaint relating to a couple and not just to a single person. Both partners should be involved in the investigation and treatment.

DEFINITIONS

- **Primary female infertility** implies that the woman has never conceived.
- **Secondary infertility** indicates that at least one previous conception has taken place
- **Infertility** is generally regarded as the inability to achieve pregnancy after one year of adequate sexual exposure. **Reproductive failure** is regarded as the repeated failure to carry a pregnancy to viability
- **"Sterility"** is the term used when an individual has a condition, a so-called absolute factor, which prevents conception. This implies that the condition is irreversible.

INCIDENCE

The incidence of infertility is approximately 15–20 percent (one in every five to six couples). The different causes of infertility are listed in Table 22.1, below.

Table 22.1 Causes and frequencies of infertility

Unexplained	3.4%
Abnormal semen	36.0%
Anovulation	29.0%
Tubal damage	57.0%
Endometriosis	4.0%
Abnormal cervical mucus	7.0%
Uterine factor	6.0%

EVALUATION

During the evaluation of a couple it is helpful to categorise the various factors involved in order to cover all areas of importance.

Table 22.2 Basic infertility evaluation

Anatomical factors	■ Vagina: Anatomical defects, infections, lubricants, psychosomatic manifestations. ■ Cervix: Anatomical defects, infections, absent or excessive mucus production, surgery. ■ Uterus: Anatomical defects, infections, surgery. ■ Fallopian tubes: Anatomical defects, infections, surgery. ■ Pelvic peritoneum: Adhesions, endometriosis, infection. ■ Ovaries: Functional disorders, infection, surgery, endometriosis.
Systemic factors	■ Pathological conditions of the hypothalamus, pituitary gland, thyroid gland, adrenal glands, cardiovascular system, liver, kidney.
Immunological factors	■ Male or female immunological factors.
Pharmacological factors	■ Opioids, antiprostaglandins, chemotherapy, antidepressants
Environmental factors	■ Smoking ■ Drugs: for example antidepressants, clomiphene citrate, drugs causing hyperprolactinaemia. ■ Previous surgery: intra-abdominal or pelvic. ■ Sexual history: this must be tactfully done once confidence between doctor and patient has been established. Dyspareunia and frigidity must be excluded. Duration of sexual exposure: did intercourse occur at regular intervals over the last year? Are both partners aware of the fertile period? The opportunity is used to inform the couple about the most fertile period, that is, 12 to 14 days before the next menstruation. ■ Various vaginal lubricants, like KY jelly as well as saliva, used to improve coital satisfaction, may interfere with sperm transport or may be spermicidal. The use of these agents should be identified. Details of any previous infertility evaluation are important, including review of basal body temperature charts, previous laboratory studies and hysterosalpingograms (HSG). (The HSG for assessing tubal patency has its limitations. There is a 75 % correlation between the findings at hysterosalpingography and laparoscopy – thus a 25 % fault factor.)

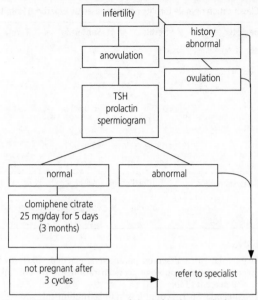

Figure 22.1 Management of the infertile couple (patient).

The investigation of the infertile couple begins with a careful history, followed by a physical examination. The interview is probably the most important part of the entire infertility investigation.

MALE INFERTILITY

Causes
Male infertility can be categorised into five aetiological groups:
- Pretesticular or pregerminal causes
- Testicular causes
- Post-testicular causes
- Genitourinary infections
- Immunological causes.

Basic semen analysis
The basic semen analysis is still the cornerstone of tests used to evaluate male fertility. The semen specimen is usually obtained by masturbation and must be collected after two to three days of abstinence to standardise the SA in all patients.

Table 22.3 Classification of male fertility potential used at Tygerberg Hospital

Semen parameter	Infertile	Subfertile	Fertile
Concentration (× 10⁶/ml)	<2.0	<15	>15
Motility (% motile)	<10	<30	>30
Forward progression (0-4)	<1.0	1.0–1.9	>2
Motility index	<20.0	20.0–49.9	>50
Morphology (% normal)	<5	<5	>5
Volume (ml)	<1.0	<1.5	>1.5
MAR test	>50%	>50%	<50%

Fertile: optimal chance for conception	**Infertile**: very small chance for conception
Subfertile: reduced chance for conception	**Sterile**: azoospermia or globozoospermia

DEFINITIONS

- **Normospermia**. Normal semen parameters, ejaculate likely to be fert (>5 percent normal morphology), concentration >15 million/ml, moti percent >30 percent (Table 22.3)
- **Oligozoospermia**. Sperm count less than 20 million/ml
- **Asthenozoospermia**. Less than 30 percent motile spermatozoa w forward progression of less than two (scale of 0 to 4)
- **Teratozoospermia**. Less than 5 percent spermatozoa with norr morphology. The Tygerberg strict criteria is now the accepted criteria by World Health Organisation in Geneva, and is the suggested internatio standard
- **Oligoastheno-teratozoospermia**. Signifies disturbance of all th variables (amount, motility, morphology). Combinations of only t parameters may also be possible
- **Azoospermia**. No spermatozoa in ejaculate
- **Globozoospermia**. Sperm with round head and no visible acrosome
- **Aspermia**. No ejaculate
- **Fertile**. Optimal chance for conception
- **Subfertile**. Reduced chance for conception
- **Infertile**. Very small chance for conception
- **Sterile**. Azoospermia or globozoospermia.

TREATMENT OPTIONS

There are many options to treat the male. A new treatment is intracytoplasmic sperm injection (ICSI.)

Micromanipulation – ICSI – (intracytoplasmic sperm injection)

Micromanipulation is a new development in the field of male infertility used for injecting selected spermatozoa into the oocyte. Indications for this treatment are: if the patient has a very low sperm count (oligozoospermia), severe asthenozoospermia, severe teratozoospermia or azoospermia. In the case of azoospermia, spermatozoa can be obtained and injected after testicular biopsy. A biopsy specimen can also be frozen in small quantities and used when required for intracytoplasmic sperm injection (ICSI) with excellent results. Thus in these cases micromanipulation (ICSI) can be applied in conjunction with IVF to try to achieve a pregnancy.

23 | Polycystic ovary syndrome

T I Siebert, T F Kruger

(See Chapter 32 in *Clinical Gynaecology*, 4th edition for more detailed information.)

Polycystic ovary syndrome (PCOS) is one of the most common endocrinopathies in women. It was first described by Stein and Leventhal in 1935.

DEFINITION

In essence, there are three major criteria, with two out of three required for diagnosis:

- Oligo- or anovulation
- Clinical and/or biochemical signs of hyperandrogenism (with the exclusion of congenital adrenal hyperplasia, Cushing's syndrome, androgen-secreting tumours, thyroid abnormalities and hyperprolactinemia)
- Polycystic ovaries on ultrasound.

PREVALANCE

A 3–11 percent prevalence of the syndrome is reported, depending on the criteria used for definition.

CLINICAL PRESENTATION

As the most common of endocrinopathies and reproductive disorders in women, it is essential that we be aware of PCOS. It is presented clinically primarily by menstrual irregularity, androgen excess (hirsutism), acne, androgen-dependent alopecia and infertility.

Table 23.1 Criteria for the metabolic syndrome in women with PCOS (three of five qualify for the syndrome)

Risk factor	Cut off
1. Abdominal obesity (waist circumference)	>88 cm
2. Triglycerides	≥150 mg/dL / ≥1.8 mmol/L
3. HDL cholesterol	<50 mg/dL / <1.3 mmol/L
4. Blood pressure	≥130/≥85 mmHg
5. Fasting and 2-h glucose from oral GTT	Fasting glucose >110-126 mg/dL or >6-7 mmol/L 2-h glucose >140-199 mg/dL or >7.8-11.1 mmol/L

DIAGNOSIS

Ultrasonography/imaging

- 12 or more follicles measuring 2–9 mm
- Increased ovarian volume (>10 cm^3).

Endocrine diagnosis

- A characteristic finding is the increase of **LH relative to FSH**. Some 50–60 percent of subjects have an elevated LH/FSH ratio, with a ratio greater than 2 : 1 being commonly accepted as consistent with PCOS
- Increased serum levels of **testosterone** (T), in particular the free T index
- **DHEAS and A4** have thus far been accepted widely as additional androgens that, like testosterone, may typically be elevated in PCOS, as reported by many investigators
- **Insulin resistance**: The HOMA index is probably the most commonly utilised formula in our clinical setting, simply calculated by the product of fasting insulin (I_0) and fasting glucose (G_0), divided by constant 22.5. A level above 2.5 is generally accepted as consistent with insulin resistance (IR). HOMA = $[I_0 \text{ (uIU/ml)} \times G_0 \text{ (mmol/L)}]$ / 22.5.

PCOS AND ANOVULATORY INFERTILITY

Methods to induce ovulation

- **Weight loss**
- **Anti-oestrogen treatment**
  Clomiphene citrate
- **Aromatase inhibitor treatment**
  The third-generation aromatase inhibitors, anastrozole and letrozole
- **Insulin sensitisers**
  Metformin
- **Gonadotropin therapy**
  Gonadotrophin therapy is often used as a second-line therapy in anovulatory women with PCOS if they were either resistant to ovulation induction with anti-oestrogen treatment or failed to conceive
- **Ovarian drilling**.

PCOS AND LATER LIFE

- The diagnosis of PCOS has serious implications not only for a woman's reproductive potential but also for her future long-term health
- In a population of women with PCOS, approximately 30 percent will develop impaired glucose tolerance (IGT) and up to 10 percent will have diabetes
- Women with PCOS are at an increased risk of an adverse cardiovascular profile

- In women with PCOS, unopposed oestrogen arising from chronic anovulation may constitute a risk factor for **endometrial hyperplasia** and **cancer**, although epidemiological evidence of links between PCOS and endometrial cancer is limited
- Despite some reports that the incidence of benign breast disease is increased in women with PCOS, this has not been confirmed and the evidence for an increased risk of breast cancer in women with PCOS is lacking.

NOTES:

24 | Endometriosis and adenomyosis

J P van der Merwe, D J Botha, T F Kruger

(See Chapter 33 in *Clinical Gynaecology*, 4th edition for more detailed information.)

Endometriosis is one of the most common gynaecological conditions affecting women of reproductive age. Although Rokitansky had recognised it as a clinical entity in 1860, its cause and pathology remain enigmatic.

DEFINITION

Endometriosis is defined as the presence of tissue, histologically similar to endometrium, at sites outside the uterine cavity. A definite histological diagnosis requires two of the three following features: endometrial glands, stroma and haemosiderin pigment. This condition is also termed "endometriosis externa".

INCIDENCE AND PREVALENCE

As making a diagnosis of endometriosis requires the use of invasive methods, the true prevalence rate can only be estimated as follows:

- General population aged 15–50: 2.5–33 percent
- Females evaluated for acute or chronic pain: 12.5 percent
- Females with localised pain, or severe dysmenorrhoea: 32 percent
- Infertile females: 30 percent.

AETIOLOGY (HISTOGENESIS)

The mechanism by which the development of endometriosis occurs is unknown and there is much discussion as to the origin of the aberrant endometrial cells. The main theories are those listed below.

- Transplantation of shed endometrium
- Retrograde menstruation
- Lymphatic and haematogenous dissemination
- Iatrogenic dissemination
- Coelomic metaplasia
- Activation of embryonic cell rests
- Familial and genetic factors
- Menstrual factors
- Delayed childbearing
- Outflow obstruction

- Hormones
- Immunological factors.

CLINICAL PRESENTATION

Endometriosis most commonly occurs within the pelvis – on or within the ovaries, on the peritoneum, or beneath the serosa of pelvic viscera. The most frequent symptoms of genital tract endometriosis are as follows:

Table 24.1 The most frequent symptoms of genital tract endometriosis

Symptom	Likely frequency (percentage)
Dysmenorrhoea	60–80
Pelvic pain	30–50
Infertility	30–40
Dyspareunia	25–40
Menstrual irregularities	10–20
Cyclical dysuria/haematuria	1–2
Dyschesia (cyclic)	1–2
Rectal bleeding (cyclic)	1

The clinical presentation depends on the location of the disease. However, the symptoms do not correlate directly with the extent of the disease.

DIAGNOSIS

Bimanual examination
This may reveal tender uterosacral ligaments, a "cobblestone" or "shotty" felt in the pouch of Douglas, tender nodules, a thickened rectovaginal septum, a retroverted and fixed uterus, generalised or localised pelvic tenderness and/or enlarged tender ovaries.

Ovarian tumour-associated antigen (CA 125)

Ultrasonography
It may be of great assistance in confirming the presence, and especially in measuring the size, of an ovarian endometrioma.

Laparoscopy

CLASSIFICATION OF ENDOMETRIOSIS

A scheme, designed and approved by the ASRM, enables uniform and objective description of the different forms of clinical presentation and degrees of severity.

It is based on the natural progression of the disease, with considerations made for unilateral or bilateral involvement, differentiation between superficial and invasive (deep) endometriosis of the peritoneum or ovaries (or of both), and stratification for severity as minimal (Stage I), mild (Stage II), moderate (Stage III) or severe (Stage IV), as well as quantification of tubo-ovarian adhesions. The ASRM revised classification is shown in Figure 33.4 in *Clinical Gynaecology*, 4th edition.

TREATMENT OF ENDOMETRIOSIS

Surgical treatment
This can be accomplished by:
- Laparoscopy: today, the preferred method
- Laparotomy
- A total abdominal **is not always a cure** for severe endometriosis, for example if bowel infiltration is the main problem, this area must be addressed when disease/endometriosis is removed. (See chapter on Endometriosis for more detail).

Medical treatment
Several medical treatments of endometriosis have been tried:
- Nonsteroidal anti-inflammatory drugs (NSAIDs)
- Oestrogen-progestogen combination: cyclic, continuous
- Progestogens: injectable, oral
- Antiprogestins
- Gonadotropin-releasing hormone agonists (GnRHa)
- GnRHa with add-back
- Others.

MALIGNANT TRANSFORMATION IN ENDOMETRIOSIS

Malignant degeneration of an endometrial ovarian cyst may occur, but it is rare.

ADENOMYOSIS

Adenomyosis is characterised by endometrial glands and stroma being located randomly within the myometrium at a depth of more than 3 mm or two low-power fields below the endomyometrial junction.

Incidence
Because of the varying definitions, the incidence of adenomyosis may vary enormously. The mean incidence lies at 20 percent.

Symptoms
Not all patients with adenomyosis are symptomatic; about 35 percent are asymptomatic. The most frequent symptoms are:

- Menorrhagia: 50 percent
- Dysmenorrhoea: 30 percent
- Metrorrhagia: 20 percent
- Dyspareunia: occasionally.

The frequency and severity of symptoms correlate with the extent of adenomyosis. Possible reasons for the menstrual dysfunction include the following:

- Inability of the uterus to contract properly
- Greater endometrial surface area
- Prostaglandin imbalance – as mefenamic acid administration can reduce blood loss.

Diagnosis
The clinical diagnosis of adenomyosis is only suggestive at best (50 percent), and most often is either not made or over diagnosed.

- Transvaginal ultrasound scanning (TVS) seems to be of diagnostic value with a sensitivity of 87 percent, a specificity of 98 percent, a positive predictive value of 74 percent and negative predictive value of 99 percent
- The best radiological means so far is MRI, although experience is limited.

Treatment
Treatment depends on the severity of symptoms and on the patient's desire to extend her family or her unwillingness to have a hysterectomy.

Medical treatment
There is a lack of information on the specific effects of drug therapy on adenomyosis. Drugs used in the treatment of adenomyosis are mostly the same as those used for endometriosis.

Surgery
- **Laparoscopic resection** is indicated only for the well-defined adenomyoma
- **Laparoscopic myometrial electrocoagulation** is performed only by an expert in this field and for specific indications
- **Myometrial excision**. Adenomyosis may be excised if it does not involve the major portion of the uterus
- **Subtotal hysterectomy**
- **Total abdominal hysterectomy or vaginal hysterectomy**. Depending on the clinical situation, the only specific treatment may be a hysterectomy.

25 | Contraception

P S Steyn

(See Chapter 34 in *Clinical Gynaecology*, 4th edition for more detailed information.)

There are several methods of fertility control, most of them applicable to women.

BARRIER METHODS

The male condom
- The condom made of latex is one of the most commonly used methods of contraception
- Oil-based lubricants should never be used as they can damage the latex.

The female condom
The female condom (Femidom) is manufactured from polyurethane. It is a sac with a wide ring that fits over the introitus, and with a loose inner ring that fits over the cervix. This device is less likely to rupture, is resistant to chemicals and can be used without the male having a full erection. The Pearl Index with correct use is between 5 and 15.

HORMONAL CONTRACEPTION

The oral contraceptive pill
Millions of women have taken the oral contraceptive pill since the first clinical report that a combination of oestrogen and progesterone suppresses ovulation.

Different oral contraceptive pills and their effectivity
Combination pill
All these consist of a combination of an oestrogen and a progestogen (Table 25.1).

The progestogen-only pill
Each pill contains only progestogen. There are no oestrogen-containing pills and no breaks in the cycle.

Contra-indications
Absolute contra-indications to COC use
There are very few absolute contra-indications. These should be weighed against the desire to prevent pregnancy and the acceptability or reliability of

Table 25.1 Percentage of women experiencing an unintended pregnancy during the first year of typical use and the first year of perfect use of contraception and the percentage continuing use at the end of the first year. USA. (Trussel 2007, WHO MEC 2009)

Method	% of women experiencing an unintended pregnancy within the first year of use		% of women continuing use at one year
	Typical use	Perfect use	
No method	85	85	
Spermicides	29	18	42
Withdrawal	27	4	43
Fertility awareness methods	25		51
a) Standard days method*		5	
b) Two day method #		4	
c) Ovulation method #		3	
Condom (Male)	15	2	53
Combined pill and progestogen only pill	8	0.3	68
Combined hormonal patch (Evra®)	8	0.3	68
Combined hormonal ring (Nuvaring®)	8	0.3	68
Depo medroxyprogesterone acetate, DMPA (Depo-Provera®)	3	0.3	56
Combined injectable (Lunelle®)	3	0.05	56
Cu- IUCD (Copper T)	0.8	0.6	78
LNG-IUS (Mirena®)	0.2	0.2	80
Subdermal Implant (Implanon®)	0.05	0.05	84
Female sterilization	0.5	0.5	100
Male sterilization	0.15	0.1	100

* Method involves avoiding intercourse on cycle days 8–19
\# Method is based on evaluating cervical mucus

Source: Trussel J. 'Contraceptive efficacy'. In: Hatcher R A, Trussel J, Nelson A L, Cates W, Stewart F H, Kowal D. 2007. *Contraceptive Technology*, 19th rev. ed. New York: Ardent Media

other contraceptive methods. The same can be said for the relative contra-indications. It is always important to inform patients accurately about the adverse effects and contra-indications so that they can make informed decisions. Ensuring that patients can make an informed choice also reduces the prescriber's liability in case of complications.

- Pregnancy
- Uninvestigated amenorrhoea
- Undiagnosed genital tract bleeding
- Risk of arterial and venous thromboembolism (see Tables 34.5 and 34.6 in *Clinical Gynaecology*, 4th edition)
- Liver disease
  - Abnormal liver function tests
  - Gall bladder stones.
- Tumours
  - Oestrogen-dependent tumour
  - Undiagnosed genital tract bleeding.

Relative contra-indications to COC use
- Glucose intolerance
- Lactation
- Galactorrhoea which develops during pill usage
- Development of secondary amenorrhoea
- Abnormal uterine bleeding during usage
- Migraine
- Severe varicose veins
- Before a large surgical procedure.

Progestogen-only pill
The following progestogen-only contraceptives pills are available in South Africa
- Microval® levonorgestrel 30 µg
- Micro-Novum® norethisterone 35 µg.

Transdermal combined contraceptive system (Evra®)
A continuous daily serum level of 20 µg ethinyl estradiol and 150 µg norelgestromin (the primary active metabolite of norgestimate) is delivered. This is followed by a week of non-use to allow a withdrawal bleed.

Side-effects specific to the contraceptive patch include:
1. Adhesive issues related to the delivery system, although detachment rates and skin sensitivity is reported by <3 percent of users.
2. Increase in mild breast discomfort, but after the first two to three cycles, this symptom improves.
3. A potential decrease in efficacy in women weighing more than 90 kg.

Progestogen injections

Progestogens used for this purpose are **medroxyprogesterone acetate** (MPA, Depo-Provera®), and **norethisterone enanthate** (Nur-Isterate®). Deep intra-muscular administration of MPA gives contraceptive protection for three months and is the most frequent injectable form of contraception used in South Africa. Nur-Isterate® suppresses ovulation for 60 days only and must be given at two-monthly intervals.

Adverse effects
- *Irregular bleeding*: Bleeding is usually controlled by giving additional oestrogen. Ethinyl oestradiol 20–30 µg as such or any of the combined pills may be added for 21 days
- *Amenorrhoea*
- *Delayed return of fertility*
- *Weight gain*: Weight gain is seen frequently as a result of increased appetite
- *Other adverse effects*: Complaints of headache, loss of libido and depression are sometimes expressed. There is some concern over the loss of bone density in long-term users.

Contra-indications
There are very few contra-indications. They include the following:
- Pregnancy
- Undiagnosed abnormal genital tract bleeding
- Nulliparity, especially when a family is planned for the near future
- Short-term contraception
- Liver disease
- Porphyria
- Major depression.

Effectiveness
MPA is an excellent contraceptive agent as very few pregnancies are reported. The Pearl Index is 0.3.

INTRAUTERINE CONTRACEPTIVE DEVICES

Types
The intrauterine contraceptive devices (IUCDs) and systems available in South Africa offer almost complete protection from pregnancy.

Contra-indications
- Possibility of pregnancy
- Abnormal uterine bleeding
- Current genital tract infection
- Short (<5.5 cm) or distorted uterine cavity
- Heart valve prosthesis or past attack of infective endocarditis
- Dysmenorrhoea (relative contra-indication).

Complications

- *Salpingitis*: IUCDs increase the risk of salpingitis by three to five times in highrisk groups
- *Pain*
- *Lost strings*: Lost strings can indicate expulsion of the device or pregnancy.

Postcoital contraception

Postcoital contraception is also called emergency contraception. It is used to prevent unwanted pregnancy after unprotected sexual intercourse or failure of a barrier method. Three methods are available.

Table 25.2 Available methods for postcoital contraception

1   **Combined oral contraceptive regimen**: two pills each containing 50 µg ethinyl oestradiol and 250 µg levonorgestrel immediately, repeated after 12 hours. Commercially available as E-Gen-C®. This hormonal dosage is the same as in the active pills of Nordiol® and equivalent to Ovral®.
2   **Progestogen only**: levonorgestrel 0.75 mg immediately, repeated after 12 hours. Commercially available as NORLEVO®. This hormonal dosage is equivalent to 25 Microval® pills stat and 25 pills after 12 hours.
3   **A copper-containing IUCD** inserted within 120 hours of unprotected intercourse.

STERILISATION

When a woman has completed her family and she is certain that this decision is permanent, sterilisation can be considered. This is one of the most effective and most economic methods of family planning. Either the man or the woman may be sterilised, depending on various circumstances.

Female sterilisation

Before planning female sterilisation it is important to exclude any serious underlying genital tract pathology which may require operative management. Typical examples are abnormal cervical cytology or uterine pathology. Sterilisation should not be considered before the cervix and the uterus have been investigated properly and the necessity for hysterectomy has been excluded.

Patient counselling for sterilisation must include the following:
- The finality of the procedure
- Alternative available methods

- Discussion about possible consequences, complications and implications:
  - patients should not be forced into a decision, especially during labour or when stress or confusion influences their emotional status, as this may lead to feelings of regret, guilt and sexual dysfunction
  - the procedure may fail in a small percentage of cases.

Male sterilisation
Vasectomy
Vasectomy is a simple operation that can be performed under local analgesia as an outpatient procedure. Morbidity of the operation is very low.

REVERSAL PROCEDURES
Female
Microsurgical technique or laparoscopic in some specialised units.

Success rate
Patency rate – 80-90%
Pregnancy rate after 1 year – ±60-70%

Male
Microsurgical reversal

Success rate
Patency rate – 70%
Pregnancy rate – 40-70% dependent on the duration of reversal.
A pregnancy rate of 40-60% can now be achieved after 15 years or longer post vasectomy when reversed.

SECTION 4 | Urogynaecology

26 | Disorders of the lower urinary tract

P de Jong

(See Chapter 35 in *Clinical Gynaecology*, 4th edition for more detailed information.)

The pelvic floor is a functional unit, and dysfunction can lead to urinary or faecal incontinence, pelvic pain or genital prolapse.

LOWER URINARY TRACT SYMPTOMS (LUTS)

Definitions
- **Urinary incontinence:** The complaint of any involuntary loss of urine
- **Urgency urinary incontinence** is the complaint of involuntary leakage associated with urgency
- **Stress urinary incontinence** is the complaint of involuntary leakage on effort or exertion, or on sneezing or coughing
- **Mixed urinary incontinence** is the complaint of involuntary leakage associated with urgency and also with effort, exertion, sneezing and coughing
- **Nocturnal enuresis** is any involuntary loss of urine occurring during sleep
- **Insensible urinary incontinence:** the complaint of incontinence where the woman has been unaware of how it occurred
- **Coital incontinence:** loss of urine with coitus, either with penetration or at orgasm
- **Overactive bladder (OAB)** is characterised by the symptoms of urgency with or without urgency incontinence, usually with frequency and nocturia.

EVALUATION OF THE INCONTINENT PATIENT

History and clinical examination form the basis of the approach
Special investigations:
- Urinalysis by dipstick
- Estimation of postvoid residual urine (PVR) by scan or catheterisation
- Initial imaging may be by ultrasound, or X-ray
- Cystoscopy
- Uroflowmetry.

Urodynamic testing

Table 26.1 The aims of urodynamic evaluation

- The assessment of bladder sensation
- The detection of detrusor overactivity
- The assessment of urethral competence during filling
- The determination of detrusor function during voiding
- The assessment of outlet function during voiding
- The measurement of residual urine
- The assessment of bladder compliance.

MANAGEMENT OF URINARY INCONTINENCE

Stress urinary incontinence (SUI)

The aetiology of stress urinary incontinence is poorly understood, and four groups of risk factors may be identified (Table 26.2).

Table 26.2 Risk factors for stress incontinence

Predisposing factors	■ Genetic predisposition ■ Anatomic, neurological and muscular abnormalities
Inciting factors	■ Pregnancy / childbirth / parity
Promoting factors	■ Obesity ■ Constipation ■ Lung disease and smoking (chronic cough) ■ Neurological diseases ■ Drugs / medication
Decompensating factors	■ Age ■ Dementia and debility ■ Co-morbidities and changes in environment

The most studied and proven risk factors are age, obesity and vaginal parity

Conservative management of SUI

- *Physiotherapy*
  - Of proven benefit in compliant women.
- *Devices*
  - Pessaries are generally of limited value in the treatment of incontinence.
- *Drug therapy*
  - This has very little place in the management of stress incontinence.

Surgical management of SUI

This becomes an effective option when conservative management has failed. It is important to choose the correct operation for the patient, dependent on her unique situation. Examples of operations are:

- Tension-free vaginal tape procedures (TVT)
- The Burch colposuspension if patient needs concominant laparotomy.

The overactive bladder (OAB) and urgency incontinence

- *Bladder training*

  Bladder training is a form of behaviour therapy, to help the patient regain bladder control by increasing the effective capacity of the bladder and thereby reducing the symptoms of the overactive bladder.

- *Medication*

Table 26.3 Useful drugs in the management of the overactive bladder

Drug	Dose	Notes
Oxybutinin (Ditropan)	2.5 mg bd or tds 5 mg tds maximum	Now available in daily XL form
Tolterodine (Detrusitol)	2 mg / 4 mg SR once daily	Fewer side-effects than oxybutinin
Propiverine (Detrunorm)	15 mg bd dose	Anticholinergic and spasmolytic
Trospium (Uricon)	20 mg bd	As effective as oxybutinin and tolterodine
Darifenacin (Enablex)	7.5 mg, 15 mg daily controlled release	M3 selective receptor antagonist Low CVS or CNS risk
Solifenacin (Vesicare)	5 mg/10 mg daily	Uptitrate to 10 mg to improve benefit as needed
Oestrogen	Topical vaginal use	Useful for irritative OAB symptoms and genital atrophy
Ethipramine or **imipramine**	10-25 mg bd. Begin with lowest dose	Use with caution in the elderly. Inexpensive. Useful for enuresis.

27 | Genital prolapse

G Rienhardt

ANATOMY

Muscular structures, ligaments and fascia serve as the main supports of the pelvic organs. The levator ani makes up the pelvic floor with the pubococcygeal portion being penetrated by the lower vagina and urethra. This muscle contracts and helps to maintain the position of the organs.

AETIOLOGY

Damage to the supports of the pelvic organs will predispose a patient to prolapse.

Table 27.1 Causes of genital prolapse

A. CONGENITAL
Connective tissue disease

B. CHILDBIRTH
Large babies
Prolonged labours
Instrumental deliveries

C. IATROGENIC FACTORS
Poor hysterectomy technique
Retropubic bladder neck suspension

D. CONDITIONS CAUSING RAISED INTRA-ABDOMINAL PRESSURE
Chronic respiratory disease
Pelvic masses
Obesity
Chronic constipation.

Table 27.2 Symptoms of prolapse

A. GENERAL
Pressure
Protrusion of lump
Dragging sensation
Coital difficulty
Backache
Difficulty walking
Ulceration, bleeding, discharge.

B. ANTERIOR WALL PROLAPSE
Urinary stress incontinence
Urinary retention/incomplete emptying
Recurrent urinary tract infection
Poor stream
Frequency, urgency.

C. POSTERIOR WALL PROLAPSE
Constipation
Incomplete bowel emptying
Vaginal/perineal splinting
Digitation after defecation.

Table 27.3 Classification of prolapse

A. ANTERIOR COMPARTMENT
Urethrocele (urethra, bladder neck)
Cystocele (bladder).

B. MIDDLE COMPARTMENT
Uterine prolapse (uterus)
Vault prolapse (vaginal vault after hysterectomy).

C. POSTERIOR COMPARTMENT
Rectocoele (lower rectum)
Enterocoele (small bowel/omentum).

CLINICAL EXAMINATION

- Prolapse is a clinical diagnosis
- Simple prolapse refers to prolapse in one compartment only
- Complex prolapse involves more than one compartment
- The Sims speculum is the instrument of choice in the examination of prolapse.

For clinical use, a simple and practical grading of prolapse is available. It is summed up in Table 27.4.

Table 27.4 Grading of prolapse

Grade 1	Descent within the vagina, but not to the introitus.
Grade 2	Descent down to, but not through the introitus.
Grade 3	Descent through the introitus.

Special investigations
These are usually unnecessary because the diagnosis is made on clinical grounds. Patients with concomitant urinary or bowel complaints should be referred for additional investigations. These could include cystometry, anal manometry, transanal ultrasound and electrophysiological studies. Urine culture and cervical cytology should be checked. Any pelvic mass must be appropriately investigated.

Differential diagnosis
There are other masses which may present at the introitus and could be mistaken for prolapse.

Masses arising from the urethra and vagina
- Polyp
- Vaginal leiomyoma
- Urethral caruncle
- Urethral diverticulum
- Paraurethral cyst
- Urethral mucosal prolapse.

Uterine masses
- Prolapsed leiomyoma
- Prolapsed endometrial polyp
- Cervical polyp
- Cervical elongation (elongatio colli).

MANAGEMENT
Conservative management
- Hormone replacement therapy
- Pelvic floor exercises
- Vaginal pessaries.

Surgery

This is the only potentially permanent remedy available. There is still a 25–30 percent chance of a recurrence of prolapse occurring, even after successful surgery. No technique has been shown to be completely effective.

Operations for various types of prolapse
Anterior compartment prolapse

- Anterior repair or anterior colporrhaphy.

Posterior compartment prolapse

- **Rectocoele repair**. The posterior repair or posterior colporrhaphy aims to repair the fascial defect and damage to the rectovaginal septum
- **Enterocoele repair**.

Middle compartment prolapse

- **Uterine prolapse**. This lends itself to **vaginal hysterectomy** with suspension of the vault from the uterosacral/transverse cervical ligament complex. Often this procedure is combined with **an anterior and posterior repair** because of multicompartment prolapse. Uterine prolapse in a younger patient wishing to have more children is best treated with hysterosacropexy. Here, synthetic mesh is attached to the back of the cervix through a suprapubic approach, and fixed to the sacral promontorium.
- **Vaginal vault prolapse**. The procedure of choice in this condition – particularly in the sexually active patient – is the transabdominal sacrocolpopexy.
- **Colpocleisis**. This is performed in frail, elderly patients who are not sexually active. It involves occlusion of the vaginal lumen by approximating the anterior and posterior vaginal walls after cutting away part of the epithelium.

28 | Gynaecological fistulae

J A van Rensburg, L Juul

(See Chapter 38 in *Clinical Gynaecology*, 4th edition for more detailed information.)

DEFINITION

- A fistula is an abnormal passage or communication between two or more internal organs or between the body surface and one or more internal organs or structures.

INCIDENCE

- The incidence varies, but the World Health Organisation (WHO) quotes the incidence as 0.3 percent for obstetrical fistulae.

AETIOLOGY AND PATHOGENESIS

Genitourinary fistulae
Obstetrical fistulae
- Neglected obstructed labour
- Obstructed labour of long duration
- The typical patient at risk for obstetric fistulae due to obstructed labour, is young (probably in her teens), primiparous, short (less than 150 cm tall), uneducated and delivers at home with no skilled attendant present
- Also, incisions in labour from poorly trained health attendants, especially in cases of female cultural circumcision, have been implicated in obstetric fistulae
- The bladder may be damaged during Caesarean section, especially if densely adherent to the lower uterine segment.

Surgical fistulae
- Risk factors for postoperative urogenital fistulae include anatomical distortion, abnormal tissue adhesion, impaired vascularity and compromised healing
- The risk for VVF is 0.1 percent after hysterectomy, almost 1 percent after laparoscopic assisted vaginal hysterectomy and 1–4 percent for radical hysterectomy. This can also occur with anterior colporrhaphy
- The incidence of ureterovaginal fistulae following radical hysterectomy for invasive cervical carcinoma is less than 1 percent.

Other
- Advanced cervical carcinoma and radiation.

Genitointestinal fistulae
Obstetrical fistulae
- 88 percent RVF occur after third- and fourth-degree perineal lacerations
- Also when an episiotomy is performed, or when a suture is placed into the rectum.

Surgical fistulae
- Unrecognised injury to the rectum at the time of posterior colpoperineorrhaphy.

Other
- Chronic granulomatous disorders. Crohn's disease is the second most common cause for RVF
- Rarely, a colovaginal fistula can develop due to the unusual complication of diverticulitis
- Large rectal or vaginal carcinomas can also lead to rectovaginal fistulae through direct invasion
- Spontaneous RVFs have been described in HIV-positive patients
- Finally, rectovaginal fistulae can occur as a result of sexual assault.

CLINICAL FEATURES AND EVALUATION
Genitourinary fistulae
- The most important symptom is urinary incontinence (UI).

On clinical examination:
- The fistula can usually be visualised if large enough
- Obstetric fistulae are frequently situated in the midvagina, whereas post-surgical fistulae can be localised high in the vaginal vault
- With the detected or suspected fistula the following main principles of investigation apply:
  - to confirm the discharge is urine
  - to establish that the leakage is extraurethral rather than urethral
  - to establish the site of leakage
  - to exclude multiple fistulae
- The bladder is filled with sterile water containing one ampoule of methylene blue, and the patient is then observed for leakage of the dye. Direct vision with the Sims speculum is preferred. If clear urine leaks the ureter is involved. With no leakage a small fistula needs to be excluded. A tampon is inserted in the vagina and the patient walks for 15–30 min. If the tampon stains, the diagnosis is confirmed

- Cystoscopy:
    - will demonstrate the location and size of the fistula
    - the ureteral orifices can be localised in relation to the fistula, and
    - a biopsy can be taken if indicated
- Intravenous pyelography is essential to detect possible ureteric involvement
- A retrograde pyelogram is more reliable to identify the exact site of an ureterovaginal fistula
- Computerised tomography is becoming increasingly more useful for the diagnosis of fistulas.

Genitointestinal fistulae
- Leakage of mucus, flatus and faeces from the rectum into the vagina
- Low rectovaginal fistulae can easily be seen on examination
- Rectal examination is essential with assessment of the integrity of the anal sphincter
- Endoultrasound is the investigation of choice to evaluate the integrity of the internal and external sphincter
- However, if the cause of the fistula is obstetric or traumatic, no additional investigations are required
- In the case of enterovaginal fistulae careful evaluation of the entire intestinal tract is indicated, and a surgeon should be consulted.

TREATMENT
- It is important to consider biopsy of fistulae in order to exclude a neoplasm or chronic granulomatous disorders.

Genitourinary fistulae
- Gynaecological fistulae are most commonly repaired surgically and referred to a centre with the necessary expertise
- Obstetrical fistula is commonly left for 2–3 months before surgical repair
- The immediate management includes continuous transurethral catheterisation for at least one month and antibiotics to control infection
- With surgical fistulae the same principles apply, but if the injury is detected within the first 24 hours immediate repair is appropriate
- In radiation fistulae the waiting period can be as long as one year
- Fistulae involving the ureters frequently require complicated urological procedures.

Genitointestinal fistulae
- The repair of rectovaginal fistulae requires bowel preparation, including the use of antibiotics. It is critical to evaluate the degree of faecal incontinence
- The technique should stick to the same principles as in the VVF flap splitting repair
- If required the sphincter must be dissected and repaired separately. A temporary diversion colostomy is rarely required as an adjunct to the repair.

29 | Puberty

T F Kruger, E Viljoen

(See Chapter 24 in *Clinical Gynaecology*, 4th edition for more detailed information.)

DEFINITION

Puberty in the female is the phase of development that begins with the onset of secondary sexual development and ends when ovulation occurs. During secondary sexual development, the sex organs mature and reproductive capacity is attained.

The pubertal events are summarised in Table 29.1.

Table 29.1 Summary of pubertal events

■ Breast budding	9.8 years -10.5 years
■ Onset of pubic hair development	10.5 -11years
■ Maximal body growth (growth spurt)	11.4 years
■ Menarche	12.8 years
■ Adult breast development	14.6 years
■ Adult pubic hair development	13.7 years

POINTS TO REMEMBER ABOUT PUBERTY AND GROWTH

- Linear growth acceleration is the first somatic sign of puberty.
- Although the sequence may be reversed, adrenarche usually appears after the breast bud with axillary and pubic hair growth 2 years later. (Table 29.1)
- The growth peak occurs about 2 years after breast budding and 1 year before menarche.
- In approximately 20 percent of children pubic hair growth may be the first sign of puberty.
- Gonadotrophins rise moderately before 10 years. This is followed by a rise in estradiol. LH pulses initially increase only during sleep but later occur throughout the day.
- Gonadal oestrogen is responsible for secondary female characteristics, vaginal and uterine growth. Skeletal growth rapidly increases as a result of low levels of gonadal oestrogen in early puberty.

- Adrenal androgen causes pubic and axillary hair growth. Adrenarche plays little or any part in skeletal growth, and is functionally an unrelated event to gonadarche, even though they are temporarily parallel.
- At midpuberty, sufficient gonadal oestrogen causes endometrial proliferation and gives rise to the first menstruation.
- In the postmenarche, cycles are anovulatory. Ovulation requires sustained, predictable LH response to estradiol which is usually only acquired in late puberty.

PRECOCIOUS PUBERTY

Definition

A girl may be considered sexually precocious if she shows signs of secondary sexual development before the age of eight years or begins to menstruate before the age of nine. Precocious puberty is five times more common in girls than in boys.

Aetiology

Precocious puberty can be due to increased gonadotropins (true precocity or GnRH-dependent precocious puberty) or due to increased sex steroids (precocious pseudopuberty or GnRH-independent precocious puberty).

Reasons for GnRH-dependent precocious puberty (true precocity) can be idiopathic, cerebral conditions and ectopic gonadotropin production.

Reasons for GnRH-independent precocious puberty (precocious pseudopuberty) are ovarian cysts/tumours, McCune-Albright syndrome, adrenal feminising tumours or adrenal masculinising tumours.

Seventy-four percent of all precocious puberty cases are idiopathic. It is, however, still of importance to rule out slowly developing lesions and thus to follow these patients over a prolonged period of time. Eleven percent is due to ovarian cysts, 7 percent due to cerebral tumours and 5 percent due to McCune-Albright syndrome. The clinician must always rule out a serious disease process of central or peripheral origin. Children presenting with precocious puberty under the age of four have a higher risk of a CNS lesion.

Diagnosis

History

First of all a thorough history and a physical examination are necessary. Furthermore, it is essential to rule out life-threatening diseases, for example neoplasm of the CNS, ovary and adrenal gland. An important question is whether the disease is still in progress or has stabilised. It is also important to remember that non-endocrinological causes of vaginal bleeding must be excluded (injuries, foreign bodies, trauma, sexual assault, oestrogen intake). Familial occurrence makes certain diseases unlikely, that is, tumours.

Physical examination

Growth, Tanner stages, height and weight percentiles must be recorded. External genitalia must be examined for any changes. Abdominal, pelvic and neurological examinations must be performed. Signs of androgenisation must be recognised. Special findings like McCune-Albright and hypothyroidism must be reported.

Special investigations

- Biochemistry:
  - FSH, LH, thyroid function tests (TSH and FT_4), β-hCG, α-FP
  - DHEAS, testosterone, oestradiol, progesterone, 17α-hydroxyprogesterone
  - Inhibin levels
  - Provocative tests: GnRH, possibly ACTH stimulated 17-OH-P.

- Imaging:
  - Wrist radiograph for bone age
  - Ultrasonography of abdomen and pelvis (ovaries, adrenals, liver)
  - CT brain or MRI (cranial, adrenals), EEG.

Treatment

Aim

- Diagnose and treat intracranial disease;
- Arrest maturation until normal puberty age, use GnRH agonist;
- Attenuate and diminish established precocious characteristics;
- Maximise eventual adult height;
- Facilitate the avoidance of abuse and reduction of emotional problems, and provide contraception if necessary.
- The drug with which the greatest experience has been gained is medroxyprogesterone acetate (MPA). It is usually administered in a dose of 100-200 mg IM weekly. This drug can slow down breast and genital development. It is not successful in reducing the accelerated growth rate and skeletal maturation.
- GnRH agonists are currently the most effective treatment of central precocious puberty.

Special conditions to remember: Premature menarche. Isolated premature menarche without other evidence of maturation is an exceedingly rare presentation of precociousness. Infection, the presence of a foreign body, abuse and trauma, and local neoplasms should be considered. Normal growth, development and fertility are not affected.

DELAYED PUBERTY

When is puberty delayed?

It is abnormal for a girl not to have any signs of secondary sexual development by the time she has reached her 14th birthday. If there is no development at the age of 14, something is wrong and investigations need to be performed. On the other hand, if a 14-year old presents with normal sexual development (complete development for more than one year) and has not menstruated yet, she may also have an abnormality, such as congenital absence of the vagina or the androgen insensitivity syndrome. Most girls have their menarche 2.3 years after the first sign of breast development.

Causes of delayed puberty

Delayed puberty occurs in 43 percent of cases due to hypergonadotropic hypogonadism, in 31 percent due to hypogonadotropic hypogonadism (18-20 percent reversible and 11-13 percent irreversible), and in 18 percent due to congenital abnormalities of the genital tract (eugonadism) (Table 29.2).

Table 29.2 Causes of delayed puberty

Hypergonadotropic hypogonadism (43%) (low oestrogen – delayed puberty)	Hypogonadotropic hypogonadism (31%) (low oestrogen – delayed puberty)	Eugonadism (normal oestrogen – delayed menarche)
Ovarian failure – normal karyotype Autoimmune 46XX gonadal dysgenesis	**Reversible (18–20%):** Physiologic delay Weightloss/anorexia Primary hypothyroidism CAH Cushings Prolactinoma	**Müllerian duct agenesis (14%)** Congenital absence of uterus and vagina
Ovarian failure – abnormal karyotype Turner syndrome 46XY gonadal dysgenesis Swyer syndrome *Streak gonads carries a high risk of malignancy and should be removed*	**Irreversible (11–13%):** GnRH deficiency Hypopit Congenital CNS defects CNS tumours Post-surgical hypopituitarism	**Uterovaginal plate (3%)** Complete vaginal septum Imperforate hymen **Intersex disorders (1%)** That is androgen insensitivity **Inappropriate positive feedback (7%)** **Chronic anovulation** PCOS – may present with delayed menarche